JEAN WATSON and
MARIE CLAYTON

Caring:
a passage
to
Heart

An anthology of
Caritas Processes®
experienced

LOTUS
LIBRARY

CARING: A PASSAGE TO HEART
An anthology of Caritas Processes® experienced

First published in Great Britain in 2020 by Lotus Library

A CIP catalogue record for this book is available from the British Library.

ISBN 978-0-5787692-9-5

Managing Editor for Lotus Library: Julie Watson
Developmental Editor: Jennifer Watson Ervedosa
Cover Design and typesetting by Clare Connie Shepherd
www.clareconnieshepherd.com
Internal illustrations ©Julie Watson www.saatchiart.com/juliewatson
image on page xi inspired by www.thebirthposter.com

Lotus Library is an imprint of Watson Caring Science Institute, a 501C(3) international non-profit foundation.

Watson Caring Science Institute, 4450 Arapahoe Avenue Suite 100, Boulder, CO 80303 USA
www.watsoncaringscience.org

LOTUS
LIBRARY

Watson Caring
Science Institute

JEAN WATSON and
MARIE CLAYTON

Caring: a passage to Heart

An anthology of
Caritas Processes®
experienced

LOTUS
LIBRARY

Table of Contents

Caritas Process 3

Caritas Process 4

Caritas Process 5

Caritas Process 6

Caritas Process 7

Authentic Caring Leadership:

Caritas Process 8

Caritas Process 9

Caritas Process 10

About This Book

The collection in this book originated from participants
taking a free online course entitled 'Caring Science
Mindful Practice' facilitated by Kathleen Sitzman.

*In 2015 when I offered the first Caring Science, Mindful
Practice Massive Open Online Course (MOOC), I didn't
know if anyone would come, or if anyone would want to share
Caritas moments from their own experiences in a public forum.
Through the process of teaching this course, I have learned that
people in nursing, allied health, and beyond; experience support,
companionship, fulfillment, validation, encouragement, and
inspiration through sharing their own unique Caritas moments and
reading those of others within this global caring community that
continues to grow each time the course is offered. I hope the caring
moments described in this book will inspire and encourage readers as
they travel their own unique caring paths.*

Kathleen Sitzman

Kathleen Sitzman, PhD, RN, CNE, ANEF, FAAN
Distinguished Watson Caring Science Scholar
Professor, East Carolina University College of Nursing

Find out more at: www.watsoncaringscience.org

caritas

ca·ri·tas

noun.

The definition of caritas is Latin
and means love for all.

Preface

Jean Watson

Living Caritas in Virtual World

An Experiential-Empirical Collection of Caritas Processes®

'Living Caritas' – a way of knowing/being/ doing/becoming, is alive and flourishing in this collection of Caritas experiences shared by global participants of Dr. Kathleen Sitzman's Massive Open Online Course (MOOC): Caring Science, Mindful Practice. Each individual narrative reveals a personal or professional truth about one of the Watson 10 Caritas Processes® – the core of the Theory of Human Caring (Watson, 1979, 1988, 2008, 2018).

These stories cross and transcend cultures, roles, professions, borders and boundaries in locations around the world. The Caritas stories and shared experiences unite us in our humanity, across time and space, congruent with an online virtual world of today, whereby space connects, rather than separates. This collection is a clear reminder that our caring consciousness transcends time, space and physicality; pointing toward a new awakening of a global phenomenon of unity through shared caritas consciousness, making new connections between caring and peace.

It is evocative and affirming to attach each story to a specific Caritas Process. I am struck as I am sure the reader will be, to what extent these narratives intersect across multiple Caritas Processes, and we invite the reader to reflect on the ways in which the whole is in the part and the part is in the whole. It is also evident, for those already familiar with the Caritas Processes, that they too overlap and intertwine with each other – creating somewhat of a gestalt – or a hologram. The whole Caritas Consciousness of each Caritas Process is contained *in a single caring moment*, and each individual Caritas Process is contained in the whole. As you enter these exemplars of Caritas, you are invited to vicariously experience each Caritas Process yourself, as each one touches and opens up our hearts to the beauty of these lived experiences of human caring/healing.

This collection invites us to enter the new territory of a virtual global caring community – moving from

Caritas to Communitas. Leibniz, the 19th century German philosopher and psychologist, envisioned a community of minds, perhaps anticipating the current web and online relationships (Watson, 2002). The shift for our time toward virtual digital worlds, is a unique time to introduce and co-create global Caritas/Communitas networks. These efforts help us to realize how to unite nurses and others across space and time to contribute to a new order of mind-to-mind (Caritas) consciousness connection in a world of cyberspace.

In an academic context, congruence between each person's experience and a specific Caritas Process can be considered a form of empirical validation of the Theory of Human Caring and real life-living experiences of Caritas. Locating each individual experience within a single Caritas Process is one way to reveal the accuracy and intersubjective confirmability of that specific Caritas Process. As we engage with these Caritas stories, we are contributing to an evolutionary leap leading to a union of technology and human consciousness for a new transpersonal reality, again whereby space connects rather than separates.

This collection is a tribute to Dr. Sitzman and her visionary passion for Caring in the Digital World as we enter a new phase in human history. Likewise, this work is a testimony to Marie Clayton and the volunteer faculty MOOC Team, who continue to offer this global virtual caring course as a form of devotion to Caritas for One Heart/One World.

Jean Watson, PhD, RN, AHN-BC, FAAN, LL (AAN)

Founder/Director Watson Caring Science Institute Boulder, Colorado USA

Distinguished Professor Dean Emerita University of Colorado Denver, College of Nursing

Recipient of 15 Honorary Doctorates (12 International) American Academy of Nursing Living Legend - 2013

References

Watson, J. (1988). *Nursing: Human science and human care.*
NY: National League for Nursing. (Rev. ed. 2008.
MA: Jones and Bartlett).

Watson, J. (2002). *Metaphysics of virtual caring communities.*
International Journal for Human Caring, 6(1), 41- 45.

Watson, J. (2008). *Nursing: The philosophy and science of
caring.* Rev. ed. Boulder, CO: University Press of
Colorado.

Sitzman, K. & Watson, J (2017). *Watson's caring in the
digital world: A guide for caring when interacting,
teaching, and learning in cyberspace.* NY: Springer.

Watson, J. (2018). *Unitary caring science: The philosophy
and praxis of nursing.* Louisville, CO: University
Press of Colorado.

Editor's Foreword

Marie Hart Clayton

Caring: A Passage to Heart
An Anthology of Caritas Processes Experienced

The aim of this book is to give you the experience of Caritas. I have been blessed to encounter the caring journey of others from what they share in the Caring Science, Mindful Practice (CSMP) course where I have been involved as a facilitator since its inception in 2015. Participants just need a device and internet access to take part in this Massive Open Online Course (MOOC). Students have the opportunity to delve deeply into Watson's 10 Caritas Processes®, mindfulness, and professional caring practices as part of the curriculum. The healing that they encounter along the way is perhaps the most compassionate support you will find anywhere in cyberspace.

I have been blessed to gather the narratives of these students and it came to me that their richness deserved a broader platform. Also because, the concepts of caring can seem abstract at times. Having relatable examples inspires us to strengthen who we are and who we are still trying to become. Indeed, the ability to see Caritas in everyday encounters may help one to begin or continue new practices.

Pure loving intentions are a hallmark of youth. I would like this book to be shared with younger audiences so that they may begin to identify and relate to Caritas. This will give them the tools they need to keep their caring core strong throughout their lives and professions.

I first met Dr. Kathleen Sitzman, the course convenor of CSMP, when I was, "knee high to a grasshopper," as she likes to say. I had just received my RN in 2003, entering a separate Bachelors degree nursing program a few weeks later. Kathy taught a Nursing Theory course, and it was here I first heard of Dr. Jean Watson and the Theory of Human Caring. Becoming a nurse had been very intentional for me. It was a calling, but more than that was my deep desire to be impactful to many people. To help them to feel the love and support we have from what many call God, Allah; I call Heavenly Father, our sacred Source of light and being. I wish to be a window to His love. And through my growing struggles during my ADN program, I wondered if I would ever be the skilled and impactful nurse I had set out to become, without a strong theoretical core. Learning about Dr. Watson's theory was like coming home after being at an intense summer camp. This work has articulated who I have always been, and who I am continuing to become. Meeting Kathy and simultaneously being introduced to Caring Theory, made me certain I was on the right path. A few years later, I had the opportunity to study with Kathy again and we have been inseparable in heart and intention ever since.

People are hungry to strengthen their core values, and are compelled to discover how to give a voice to what it is they do, and who they are, that strengthens humanity. It is thus with deep gratitude to Dr. Kathleen Sitzman, for her ingenuity, loving discernment, and commitment. Thanks to Kathy I have been a part of this world-wide endeavor which sends ripples of love and strength across our vast planet, making us all more impactful to feel and share more love and light from our Source. It has been a sacred experience for me and fulfilling to my life's work. I am also very thankful to Jean Watson for creating the language and research that was needed to validate and articulate who we are and how we can reach and become more.

It is with great love and humility I present these compassionate accounts.

Marie Hart Clayton
May, 2020
Mountain Green, Utah

10 CARITAS PROCESSES®

1. Sustaining humanistic, altruistic values by practice of loving kindness, compassion and equanimity with self/others.

2. Being authentically present, enabling faith/hope/belief system; honoring subjective inner life world of self and others.

3. Being sensitive to self and others by cultivating one's own spiritual practices; beyond ego-self to transpersonal presence.

4. Developing and sustaining loving, trusting-caring relationships.

5. Allowing for expression of positive and negative feelings — authentically listening to another person's story.

6. Creatively problem solving, 'solution seeking' through caring process; full use of self and artistry of caring-healing practices via use of all ways of knowing/being/doing/becoming.

7. Engaging in transpersonal teaching and learning within context of caring relationship; staying within other's frame of reference — shift toward coaching model for expanded health/wellness.

8. Creating a healing environment at all levels; subtle environment for energetic authentic caring presence.

9. Reverentially assisting with basic needs as sacred acts, touching mindbodyspirit of others; sustaining human dignity.

10. Opening to spiritual, mystery, unknowns — allowing for miracles.

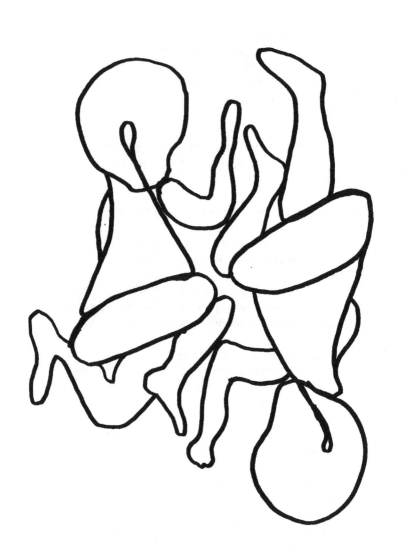

Caritas Process 1

Sustaining humanistic, altruistic values by practice of loving kindness, compassion and equanimity with self/others.

Remember What You Are Here for

Brooke Herrud RN
Sandy, Utah, USA

A profound experience I had recently in my job reminds me of Caritas Process 1. It was a Friday afternoon, and it had been a very busy day in our clinic. I was behind on scanning documents into patients' charts, completing patients' FMLA (Family and Medical Leave Act) paperwork, responding to patient messages, and helping my peers to clean up for the end of the day. Generally, I am fine with staying after work hours to complete all of these tasks, but I promised my children that I would be home on time so we could have a movie night (which meant a lot, because I have been increasingly absent at home due to heavy work loads.) I was frantic and trying to hack away at my pile of work, then a coworker came from the lobby and stated that one of our patients was crying hysterically and didn't have an appointment but wanted to be seen. The doctor I work with insisted that I go and see what she needed (as I step in with a lot of our patient care), and I was immediately panicked and somewhat irritated because of the day we had and the promise I made to my children. I took a deep breath and went out to the lobby to see what was wrong with our patient, and she stated she is newly pregnant with twins and the father of her babies just packed up and moved out. She was devastated, and the only thing that would calm her down and reassure her that everything was going to be okay was to hear the babies' heartbeats. Due to her gestational age, I was fearful that I wouldn't be able to hear the heartbeats (especially in twins). I didn't want to try to doppler her and panic her if I couldn't hear anything, so I skipped that step and grabbed an ultrasound machine so she could see her babies as well as their little flickering hearts.

I dimmed the lights for her, made sure she was comfortable, and I started scanning her belly. Tears streamed from her face as she visualized two little heartbeats on the screen, and she was relieved. I took the time to show her the tiny fingers and toes, and we watched the two little ones dance and swish around for almost an hour. She was so grateful that I took the time to reassure her that her babies were okay, especially due to the day and time of her crisis. I sincerely felt as though I needed that moment to realign myself with what my purpose is at my job. It's not so I can sit at my desk and scan papers and chart — it's so I can help women and share the love and support that I have for each and every one of them. It was such a humbling moment, and I put myself into her shoes after she left. I would've been terrified, devastated... alone. I couldn't imagine how sad and scared I would be in her situation.

This to me exemplifies Caritas 1, because what I did for this patient is not necessarily normal practice, nor is it something every patient requires. Healthcare is not one-size-fits-all, and we need to adjust as such so that our patients' individual needs are met thoroughly. I certainly did not start out in this situation with a calm and compassionate mind, but the moment I knew what I could do to help this patient to the best of my ability — I did it without question.

The Story of Bob

Jaylynn Garinger RN
Redmond, Oregon, USA

As I contemplate the first Caritas Process®, *practicing loving-kindness with self and others*, I recall an instance when I cared for a homeless patient with authentic loving-kindness. I had to be straightforward and honest with him, we had a very difficult conversation about end of life care and I believe the patient received better wholistic care because of my difficult heart to heart communication with him. We will call this homeless man Bob. He was a very frequent visitor to our emergency department. Bob was an alcoholic and had frequent struggles with pancreatitis. He also had chronic lung disease and eventually he developed terminal bladder cancer.

As his health deteriorated he was offered Hospice care, and at first he was happy to have them come and visit him in the small camp trailer where he lived. But then he was told that as a Hospice patient he could no longer request the ambulance to take him to the Emergency Room. He was very upset by this and told the hospice nurses and the social worker that if he couldn't go to the

Emergency Room when he wanted, then he no longer wanted hospice care. So, for about two months he would visit the ED two or three times a week, sometimes he would be admitted but the majority of the time he was sent home because there was really nothing the ER doctors could do for his chronic terminal conditions.

On one particular day, Bob came in on the ambulance and he was placed in one of my assigned rooms. The emergency room doctor was kind to him but bluntly told him that there was nothing the "emergency room" could do for his chronic cancer pain and the anxiety he was experiencing because of his multiple illnesses. Bob was very upset and asked me, "Why no one would help him with the problems and pain he was having?" I sat down on the stool beside his bed and looked him in his eyes. In this moment I remember being fully present for this man. I remember telling him I was sorry that he was in so much pain and that the pain and breathing problems were causing him such anxiety. I told him that I understood how having a terminal illness was not only scary, but could also cause tremendous physical pain. I further explained the doctor's reasons for not providing him with the medications he requested when he would come to the emergency room. I gently and compassionately explained that we all wanted him to have the best care possible at this time in his life and that truly this care would be best delivered by the hospice nurses. I reassured him that they could provide him with the medications he needed to be comfortable and to decrease his anxiety, and that when he needed a nurse or someone to talk with, all he would have to do is call them and someone would be out to see him that very day. I explained that the Hospice staff were all specially trained to help patients just like him in this time in their lives.

As far as I know, that was Bob's last visit to the emergency room. The next week the hospital social worker told me that Bob had asked Hospice to be involved in his care again, and a few months later Bob was able to pass away comfortably in his own space with his beloved dog at his side.

After hearing this I hoped that my intentional moments of loving-kindness and honesty with Bob, aided him in making the decision to return to Hospice care and have the best end of life care he could have received.

I know that many times the homeless and the addicts can be some of the most difficult patients to care for. In those times when, as their nurse you may become frustrated, step away, take some deep breaths and be mindful that they are human beings and they too deserve loving-kindness just like the sweet little eighty-year-old woman down the hall.

Meeting People Where They Are

Elaine Wright MSSW, PhD
Owensboro, Kentucky, USA

From my perspective as a social worker, caring professional practice means 'meeting people where they are' through the following: a) authentic engagement with the individuals and communities I serve; b) the demonstration of the values of my discipline on a micro to macro level; and c) compassion for myself, for others, and for the planet now and in the future.

I teach about Caring Theory, the ethic of care and Caritas to graduate social work students. I have the delight to witness their development of a deeper understanding of these concepts which are so self-evident in and resonant with, our professional context. Being able to explore both emotional and scientific aspects of caring, i.e. feelings and theories as part of professional practice, is both emancipatory and inspiring for them. It gives a renewed or enhanced sense of purpose and can profoundly impact their consciousness personally and professionally. As a result, they can admit, can claim, and can advocate for caring as part of being a professional practitioner.

One aspect of caring professional practice for social workers is embracing the need to more fully address how the practice of care impacts the carer, and to give more space for prioritizing self-care (for yourself and for those with whom you work). Another element is to address the potential limits or capacities for caring in a professional context. For example, can you care too much or how do you care for those who may have grossly violated the human rights of others? Acknowledging caring as part of professional practice enables a space to recognize how these situations can have an effect in the moment and over time.

Have You Had Your Mindful Moment?

Kelly Gidwani MPH, MSN, RN
Waldorf, Maryland, USA

On a day just like any other, there was a patient on our unit whose memories had failed her. She could not recall anyone's name or faces. As her dementia progressed, she couldn't even remember where she was. Each day, the nursing staff would remind her, but the longer she stayed in the hospital, the more irritated she became with this place. She began to fight with staff, and a sitter had to stay with her around the clock to keep her safe. She was fighting to be human – to be known. One day a nurse brought her a coloring page from our unit's 'Mindful Moments.' The woman's eyes lit up as she looked at all of the many shapes and the colors she could create on the page. She thanked the nurse and as they sat together, the patient became calm and focused on the sheet. They quietly connected and became centered together.

What does it mean to be human without your family nearby, helping to take care of your daily tasks or having a simple conversation? In the hospital, one's *humanness* becomes entangled in bells and whistles, and people moving about. Mindful moments create an opportunity to be human and to be known. Time taken out of the patient's day, in turn helps them become centered and participate in activities. Playing cards, coloring in a coloring book, solving a puzzle, watching the television with their nurse, or taking five minutes to have a conversation of their choosing with the clinical technician helps the patient remain uniquely themselves. This is mindful moments. Creating a space where our patients' humanity is nurtured, and where relationships between patients and nurses thrive. Everyone deserves to be known and to feel human. Have you had your mindful moment today?

Hope Through Meals and Prayers

Marie Clayton MSN, RN, Caritas Coach,
WCSI Adjunct Faculty
Mountain Green, Utah, USA

I was standing at the end of the assembly line to feed the homeless, giving bottles of water and grocery sacks to help them carry their extra fruit and utensils. I was trying to catch each person's eyes and to give them a short greeting, or wish for them to enjoy their meal, so that I could relay my loving kindness for each one.

Towards the end of the line, I saw a very thin woman approaching. I overheard her speaking about how she had end-stage ovarian cancer. She added that she was finished with her treatments as there was nothing more they could do for her. She was now facing me in line and said that she and her husband lived in a tent a few miles from here. With gratitude in her expression she told me that we couldn't imagine what coming to get these meals meant to her and her husband. This woman further affirmed for me what I do and why I do it. The life we are supporting and giving with our time distributing food is an element of service, but it is also the emotional support and shared humanity of our presence for people to know they are thought of and cared for, even by complete strangers. There is strength, hope, and energy, provided to both the giver and the receiver in choosing to nurture one another.

Pastor Jessie, who gives a short service before we serve the food, asked my 9-year-old son, Eli, to say a blessing. He told me he doesn't usually ask children to say this prayer. Eli paused as he said, "Thank you for having us be here with these... wonderful people." As a mother I was getting nervous during that pause, but I am certain my eyes were not the only ones misty from that prayer. My son could see, and everyone else was reminded of the infinite worth of each soul present that day.

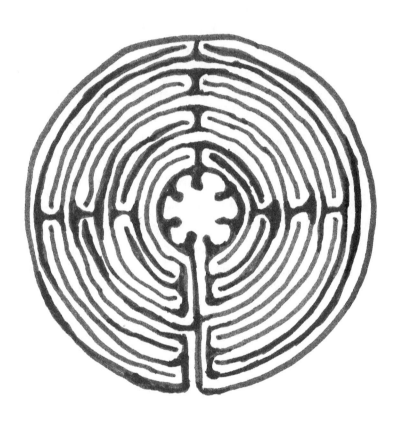

Caritas Process 2

Being authentically present,

enabling faith/hope/belief system;

honoring subjective inner life world

of self and others.

Authentic Presence is Great Love That Creates Purpose And Miracles

Dionel Venigas RN
Bocaue, Bulacan, Philippines

Based on my true life story.

Sept 25, 2019, Philippines.

Typhoon Ketsana makes landfall in our country.

The ravaging wind, days of endless rainfall, and devastating floods make their way inside the hospital first floor. There were five patients admitted to the medical-surgical floor, and only a few of us managed to clock in for work. All staff is in panic mode as we safely transfer our patients to the second floor. I am worried about my family's safety and torn between them and the call of my profession. Should I go home, braving the rain and flood? Lights start to flicker, and the feeling of anxiety and fear can be felt. I take a deep breath to calm my mind. I am here in the present moment and in this actual moment, more than the situation presents, I must channel the energy of hope and caring so that others are not alone in this current situation. I breathe out, I don't want to seclude myself in this situation. Frequent nursing rounds may be helpful. I think perhaps I'll just listen, and allow others to do the talking, just to let time pass.

During the rounds, we discussed the positive things about what life can offer after this calamity but – unexpectedly – I am learning from my patients as they open up more about their life. I become part of their shared life experience. Time passes... I am hungry, we are all hungry. I haven't changed my clothing from last night's duty and the cafeteria is closed but miracles come in an unexpected moment. One of my patients has canned foods and some extra food supplies in their room which they generously share with us. It feels like my previous act of just being present, knowing my patient interpersonally is returned with this act of kindness which makes things light and easy for all.

Time to rest and I prayed. I prayed for strength in the presence of adversity, I prayed for the safety of my loved ones, I prayed for my patients' healing. I prayed for miracles.

The next morning the flood subsided. Casualties were news on the local television, the death toll went up. I signed off, out for duty, and wished my patients a speedy recovery. I arrived at home to find our home devastated by the flood, but my family was safe and unharmed. Each moment of our life is a puzzle of mystical connection of love, fear, anger, and frustration, but Authentic Presence is great love that creates purpose and miracles.

Authentic Presence Heals Misconceptions

Megan J. Schachinger BSN, RN, HSN-BC
Warren, Michigan, USA

An experience that effectively illustrates Caritas 2, is when I was in nursing school and working as a nurse technician on a Palliative Care and Hospice floor. At the time, I was working at a Catholic hospital and I often wore a cross necklace while I worked. One day my patient was a young, Jewish woman, who was experiencing a lot of pain. She was what we would call a challenging patient. From the first moment she saw me she asked me to leave adding that a woman of my faith could not care for her. She even asked me to take down the crucifix in her room. I was immediately offended. What gave her the right to judge me like that? I decided to step back and try to fully give of myself in order to effectively care for her. I would prove to her that I would care for her well, despite our differences. With each encounter I would pause, take a breath, and say a prayer before entering the room. I would sit and talk to her, even if it was for only five minutes. Throughout the shift, she became comfortable with me and even imparted some information that we could utilize to better treat her pain. At the end of the day, she asked if I was coming back in the morning. She was disappointed when I said I would not be back. I went from getting kicked out of the room at the start of my shift, to her holding my hand, giving me a hug, and thanking me for my care by the end of my shift. She felt my respect. She felt my honor to her whole self. She felt my intentional care and attentiveness. At that time whilst in nursing school, I did not understand the impact that this experience would leave on me. I often think of that woman and send some loving kindness her way, as she allowed me to learn how to handle a 'challenging' patient with intentional, authentic presence.

The Direction of My Career

Zahra Almosawi BSN, RN
Springfield, Virginia, USA

While 'getting report' (handing over information about a patient to the next nurse on duty), a nurse told me that one of my patients was being transferred to the psychiatric unit. She told me the patient was difficult and combative and advised I stay away if possible. This sparked my curiosity. I needed to know why I had to stay away from him. This is not how nurses should be.

I knew I needed to set extra time aside to assess him closely. I went into his room with his medications. He was covered with his sheet, hiding his face. I spoke to him with a kind voice. He peeked at me with one eye. He asked if I was talking to him and I said yes, asking if I could see the rest of his face. He agreed and removed the sheet. I grabbed a chair and asked if we could chat. He was surprised and said it was the first time someone had pulled up a chair and sat down. As we spoke, I learned much more about this patient. He was a pilot who had lost his job and was involved in a difficult divorce. He had developed depression and was drinking a lot. He had gotten upset in the ED where they sedated him and labeled him "difficult." When he conversed with me he spoke with intelligence and was very polite.

I became upset and disappointed at how we were caring for this man. I asked if he had shared any of this with his doctors. He said no, as he feared they would not listen or care. I encouraged him to try talking to them. After our time together, the man began speaking to his doctors and sharing with them what he has been going through.

Everything changed for him. He began speaking with the staff and doctors and was discharged home instead of to the inpatient psychiatric unit. I felt that by authentically listening to him, and creating a safe place for him to express his feelings, I made a difference.

This experience has had a huge impact on my career. I had been searching for Nurse Practitioner schools. I couldn't decide what to do with my career. My dad has always wanted me to become a NP in cardiology, as he is a cardiologist. After this experience I decided I should be a Mental Health Nurse Practitioner. I realized that what happened to this patient could happen to others. I made a difference with this patient and maybe I could make a difference for others like him. He was just the right person to help me choose which direction to go in my career.

A Learning Experience

James Dixon III BSN, RN
Stafford, Virginia, USA

This story is about how we as nurses can exchange so much more than we think throughout a patient's stay. As a new nursing graduate there was a patient on our unit for several weeks throughout my orientation. He was a total care patient due to a spinal infection and as such I was very involved in every aspect of care throughout my orientation process. At first he was terse with the staff and requested to be alone. When I introduced myself he seemed open to the idea of having a new nursing graduate which was a surprise. We would joke and talk on and off throughout the days we spent together and we shared many stories with each other. His wife and family would visit and I learned he was a pastor prior to becoming ill. I became accustomed to his routine and started to provide him with medications prior to his asking and became faster and better versed in care every day. One day he turned to me and said "Would it be okay if I said a quick prayer for you?" What stood out in this prayer was that he was praying for me, his care giver. I accepted but did not quite understand the impact until he had finished. During his prayer he detailed the various aspects of our patient-nurse relationship and noted how he appreciated the time and forethought put into his care. It felt like that experience changed the dynamic of our relationship as patient and nurse. I realized that there was more to care than connecting IVs and cleaning. From that point on I made it a point to try and make a connection like that not only with him but with other patients as well.

The next day I saw him I took some time to sit with him to talk about how his experience at the hospital was and asked him if there was anything we could be doing better, since he had been in the hospital for so long. He smiled and told me that he did not know how long he had left but he was happy that he was here because he felt like God had put him here to let him help one more person. He smiled and told me that he was proud he had met me during his stay. From the first day he felt I was an official nurse who could accomplish anything. It was touching because I realized that he felt valued as a patient, because of the dynamics of our relationship. He taught me more than I had known at the time. I had the chance to pray with his whole family on the morning he was discharged. I felt an aura of peace and I was glad to have known him.

Approximately one month later I learned he had passed due to a recurring infection. The experiences we have with our patients shape both parties involved, through holistic and authentic interactions we can heal the spirit even when the body may be damaged.

I Picked Her Up And Held Her for A While

Ciera Wall RN

Eureka, Utah, USA

Caritas 2 is one of my favorite Caritas Processes, because it embodies what nurses do every single day! We often times see people in their worst states, in a state that makes them vulnerable and it's our job to help them. We do many things that aren't basic human needs and we have all kinds of cool knowledge about diseases, medications, etc., but we also get to help with those every day needs and show love, compassion, and encouragement while we do it. I recently started working in the NICU (Neonatal Intensive Care Unit) and I had a baby who was so upset for what seemed like no reason. She was crying and had all kinds of monitors going off because she was so angry. I knew this baby had all of her basic physical needs met, so I picked her up and held her for a while. It only took a few seconds and she settled down. I think this baby just needed to feel loved, cared for, and have someone show her compassion and the way to show this to a baby is to hold them. It's so important to remember that people have all kinds of basic needs that we can help care for. Feeling loved and cared for is a basic need and nurses are put in a place to meet this need. Nurses are put in one of the most unique positions because not only can we treat a patient medically, but we also serve to meet those emotional and mental needs when patients are struggling.

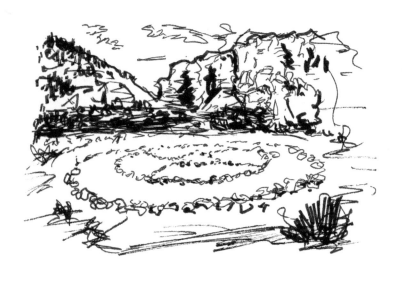

Caritas Process 3

Being sensitive to self and others
by cultivating one's own spiritual
practices; beyond ego-self to
transpersonal presence.

Meeting Michael
My Spirit Guide

Marian Turkel PhD, RN, NEA-BC, FAAN, Caritas Coach
Fort Lauderdale, Florida, USA

I was experiencing a difficult time in my personal
and professional life when I planned a trip to Sedona,
Arizona, to experience the earth's energy and the power
spots there. My mother-in-law had recently died, and
I was an Assistant Professor wondering if I would ever
be able to write or do research. Sedona is known for
Energetic Vortexes, Medicine Wheels, and Power Spots
which allow for healing. I hired a tour guide experienced
in energy work to take me to the various energy vortexes,
and to work with me to understand the power and
energy associated with the different vortexes.

We sat together inside Kachina Woman, one of the
vortexes known for healing and radiating a blue aura.
Kachina Woman represents the divine feminine. As
we sat in different vortexes, my guide asked me to set
intentions and allow the healing energy to become one
with my body. I set the intention that I want to be able to

do scholarly writing and to be open to the spiritual and unknown mystical forces of Sedona.

A few nights later, I took a UFO tour and experienced seeing many orbs of light in the night sky, a reminder that we as humans are not alone in the world.

I felt peaceful and relaxed in Sedona and I soon became comfortable going on long walks on my own. One day I ventured out alone to climb a mountain trail. The trail could only be accessed by hotel guests. While walking on the trail I saw a medicine wheel inside a cave, and I went inside to see if I could experience any energy. I remember my body tingling with a surge of energy. As I emerged from the cave and returned to the trail, I spotted a Native American park ranger dressed in ranger clothes and carrying a lunch bucket. I told him I was doing healing work and asked him his name. He told me his name was Michael, the same as my husband's name. I returned to the hotel, and the staff asked me if I had enjoyed my walk. I told them that I had met the Native American park ranger and described him. They all looked at me and said, "We do not have any Native American park rangers here." I believe Michael is my Spirit Guide and a reminder to stay grounded and connected to Mother Earth. I returned home to Florida and Florida Atlantic

University College of Nursing. My intention for writing and doing research has become a reality.

Discovering The World Within

Sara Horton-Deutsch PhD, RN, FAAN, ANEF,
Caritas Coach, Professor
San Rafael, California, USA

I recently attended a retreat on states of consciousness essential to transformation and profound awakening. We explored states of consciousness humans experience such as mystical moments where we directly glimpse the ultimate nature of reality. What struck me most profoundly was the discovery of five simple practices to recognize these experiences and their potentially transformative and healing effects. The first is to study. Through reading, reflecting, writing, and dialoguing with others, we open ourselves to the sacred, to the mind-body-spirit connection, to the mystery, to miracles, and the unknown. Second of all, is to travel. Every culture has its unique history, artifacts, foods, traditions, and ways of relating. Seeing and experiencing different cultures taps into our senses and expands our worldview. Thirdly, learn about energy work. Being sensitive to energy requires slowing down to notice. Asking ourselves, "What is going on in my mind and body at this very moment? How is it influencing my spirit?" For example, mindfulness meditation is one way to slow down and facilitate greater awareness. Remember, ultimately the Divine cannot visit us if we are not at home. Quiet, meditative states create an environment for mystical experiences to occur and for us to notice them. Next, regularly connecting with a teacher, mentor, or a community; provides a safe container to explore and continue our unique journey. Being in a community with others reminds us of our unity, helping us to recognize we are not alone, and we are ultimately all connected as one. Finally, transformation requires commitment and a radical mindset. This requires being courageous and having the willingness to lose who we think we are, and to face the unknown. To remain consistently open to self and others, always inviting mystery. These five practical principles guide our journey to higher consciousness.

Introspections On Healing Touch Experience

Judith Tipton MSN, RN, CCRN, NPD-BC

Falls Church, Virginia, USA

I have always perceived myself as being on a personal journey as a healer. I have had glimpses over the years, as I am very empathic and seek to help others. I have been on a journey to establish the most healing loving environment for myself, my family, my staff, and my patients. When I was a child of four years of age, I tried to help my neighbor friend, who was losing the battle with muscular dystrophy. My five-year-old sister and I spoke gently to him and tried to give energy to his limbs.

I have, unfortunately, helped others at times, to the detriment of my own wellbeing and resilience. My empathetic nature led me to study nursing starting in 1971. When caring for my patients and my students, where I could feel their pain, I sought to ameliorate it.

As a caring person, I thought that was what I was supposed to do. I still practiced promoting a healing loving environment. However, I was largely de-energized after more than forty years as an RN, because there seemed to be too much toxicity in my environment, and I was often, unable to rise above it.

Since coming to Inova Health, I have met a wonderful model and teacher of loving kindness. On one of the first days of my nursing orientation, she mentioned to me that there was a course on "Healing Touch" offered throughout the year. I felt compelled to purchase the book. I read it and began to practice "color chakra breathing" each morning. When I was finally able to take the course, I was amazed to learn many techniques to help others and myself! I never thought I could help myself! Since taking the class, I wake up every morning and connect my chakras. I practice a mind clearing technique throughout the day, which helps me heal myself and others. I have encouraged others to take the Healing Touch course to reap the rewards as I have done.

Since completing the course, I have had many encounters where I have mentored family, friends and staff in simple healing practices. At a skills fair I taught clinical technicians how to, "Breathe in the chakras." This provided them with energy to fuel themselves and enabled them to minister to others. I also began a journey, volunteering at the Inova cancer center where I have administered Healing Touch sessions for their clients, along with other clinicians. The positive flow of energy in the room has been transforming. I can feel and allow for the flow of this loving energy. It is amazing how cathartic and uplifting this experience has been. Healing touch has allowed me to have healthy energetic boundaries which promotes my own wellbeing and resilience.

Giving It Back To God

Melissa McElfish MA, BSN, RN, CCRN, SCRN
Sterling, Virginia, USA

We always tell our patients' family members that they need to get rest, eat, and take care of themselves, because they can't take care of their loved one if they haven't taken care of themselves. We say this every day, but as nurses, we don't often practice what we preach. In the Neuroscience ICU, we take care of critically ill patients who don't often survive. The cases that hurt the most are those that strain us ethically and morally.

I was caring for a middle-aged patient who had experienced a massive brain bleed and was progressing to brain death. I spent three days in a row counseling the family, sitting in on family meetings, explaining and re-explaining the prognosis. The family was split. One half believed that the patient, given more time, would recover as a result of a miracle. The other half understood the prognosis and believed that they should withdraw life support. The patient's daughter was the decision-maker and was torn. I found myself exhausted from everything of myself I had given this patient and family, and I was just sad about the situation. On the last shift I spent with them, they requested the chaplain, and I requested to see him when they were done.

The chaplain asked me how I dealt with these things normally. I told him I just did. I tried to compartmentalize. Eventually, I broke down. He asked me to take a walk with him. We walked to the staff exit, an elevator area between two sets of double doors with a window next to a digital time clock. "What's the last thing you do before you leave?," he asked.

"Clock out," I said.

"Now, look out the window and tell me what you see."

As I looked through the window, tears drying on my face, I told him, "Blue sky. Autumn leaves. Cars. People going about their day."

"That's the majesty of God," he said. "Every day, for twelve plus hours, you come here and you do God's work. At the end of your day, after you clock out, I want you to stand here and give it back to God. Let Him take over again for the next twelve hours, or however long until you're back. Now it's your time for you and your family, so give it back to God and go home."

I found this practice so simple and yet so profound. I implemented it into my daily nursing practice immediately. Since that day, I have never left a shift without performing this ritual. I share it with anyone who will listen. It reminds me at the end of the day to take care of myself, so that I can take care of others.

Light At The End of The Tunnel

Sharyl Eve Toscano PhD, MS, BS, RN-CPN
Anchorage, Alaska, USA

During a particularly difficult week on our unit, we experienced two expected pediatric deaths of children we had cared for, who had been on the unit for extended stays during the period of their illness. We had another unexpected infant death within one day. There were so many instances of mindful caring for these patients, however I would like to focus on how we cared for each other.

In one of these situations there existed a great deal of verbal abuse which the nursing staff sustained from both the patient and the family. We all recognized that the patterns of communication and human interactions pre-existed this new life event. Over the course of the illness nurses were present, non-judgmental, and helped this family with connection. But again, that is not the focus of this post. During this period, it was not uncommon for nurses to be seen crying at the end of their shift, or in corners during the shift. We were mindful of this experience as a group, and shared that we too were having difficulty with not only the hurtful words we were experiencing, but also the guilt we felt at having feelings about those words in the face of such a catastrophic health event for this family.

I noticed that sharing and caring allowed nurses to be present for the patient and family, whilst also being mindful and caring for self and the team. On the day of the third death, after the body had been taken for final arrangements and the family had left the unit, nurses from around the hospital came up to our unit and gathered around. They brought coffee and small snacks and their loving presence and support. This simple act of mindful caring created a lasting bond amongst all of the staff, united in one mission: to care for the population we serve.

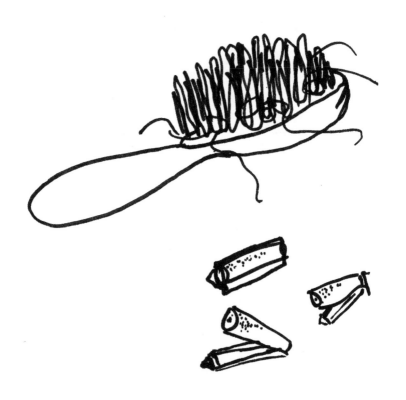

Caritas Process 4

Developing and sustaining loving,

trusting-caring relationships.

School Nursing: A Work of Heart

Angela O. Preddy RN, BSN, NBCSN

Stem, North Carolina, USA

I am a school nurse and practice in a unique setting in a rural, poverty stricken area. Being a medical professional in an educational world has its challenges, but I can honestly say through my experiences, it is the most rewarding role in my career so far. I am constantly required to think outside the box and search for answers and paths to provide for struggling families in this community. But it's such an amazing way to use my skills, to not only see immediate results, but also appreciate long term growth in my students and in their families. I not only see to their medical needs such as: practice case management, first aid and mental health... I see how real life, diversity, socioeconomic status, trauma, and family dynamics; all play a part in the health and wellbeing of a child.

Adolescence is such a fragile time for the mind and body, yet many of our children suffer immensely from trauma and medical complications like never before. Many times I feel as if I am treating the entire family, helping to build bonds, relationships and trust in order to educate, guide and care for them and their physical needs.

I have one student who has Type I diabetes. We check his blood sugar 3 times a day at school, and he also receives 4 total *Lantus* and *Novolog* injections throughout the school day. Sadly, he is only eight years old. His father died two years ago by drowning while trying to save the boy's older brother, in the local lake where many families go to enjoy the outdoors. His brother survived but tragically his father did not. His mother suffers from severe bipolar disorder and he lives with his disabled grandmother in a house they have long outgrown.

It is a daily challenge to support and educate this family, and unfortunately my sweet student has had to grow up much faster than expected by taking on the role of caring for his own diabetes mostly by himself because no one in the home truly understands the condition. There are some days he just cries and says, "I don't want to do this anymore" or, "My finger hurts!" or, "I am tired of needles." And even though as nurses we have to be strong for our patients and support them, a part of me cries inside with him. I have children the same age as him, so this makes it even more personal when I see this child having to handle such complex issues at such a young age. I don't judge because I know that, even though there are gaps, this family is doing the very best they can. I accept them for who they are.

My role in this boy's life is not only to educate and calculate doses, etc, it is also to comfort and listen because ultimately this will ease many of his fears, and promote his wellbeing. That hopefully, will last a lifetime. The rewarding part is that he knows I am here. He looks forward to seeing me, and I get to see him grow year after year here at school with me.

A caring professional practice holds within it an innate human connection that as a nurse, I get to live and breathe each day, knowing that my knowledge, skills, love, confidence and concern for my patients; will have a positive outcome not only on their health but also in their minds and hearts. To me, being able to impact someone's life on this level is what is considered "caring professional practice," and it encompasses the answer to many of my day-to-day experiences as a school health nurse. Whether I am caring for a student, staff member, or family member... I have found that **caring paves the foundation for success.** I have seen the rewards time and time again and will continue to provide this for those I care for both personally and professionally.

The Power of A Transpersonal Caring Connection – A Chief Nursing Officer's Story

Karen White-Trevino DNP, RN, NE-BC, ACHE,
Caritas Coach®
Pensacola, Florida, USA

He waited patiently, dressed in a suit and tie in the office of the hospital Chief Nursing Officer (CNO). This frail, 80+-year-old man, Mr. C was prompt in arriving for his scheduled appointment to share his recent experience at the hospital. I was the CNO, and knew this was a 'service recovery' situation.

My transition into this executive role was recent when I met with Mr. C, to hear his concern about the recent hospitalization of his wife, who had been discharged home earlier in the month. I was not emotionally prepared for his anguishing story. His wife of over sixty years, had died shortly after being discharged home from the hospital. He shared his deep sorrow. Could he have prevented this? He described his guilt. He explained how he and his wife felt voiceless when communicating with the care team during the hospitalization. The despair of this broken-spirited man was heart wrenching. I committed to him that I would share the details of the experience with the nurse leaders. In doing this, I came to realize the importance of formalizing a specific Patient & Family Centered Care Model (PFCCM) to give voice to the voiceless.

At a subsequent scheduled visit, Mr. C. returned and again, was in his formal dress attire. This time he brought a framed picture of his wife. He wanted me to have this precious picture to share with the nurse leaders so they could understand and connect with the person behind the story... The story of Mrs. C. As I accepted this gracious gift I felt my relationship with this elderly man grow stronger. His grief was still palpable, but his guilt had been reduced through deep conversation shared between us, and welcomed stories of his beautiful relationship with his loving wife.

From then on, I used the picture of Mrs. C. as the opening centering exercise for every nurse leadership meeting. A reminder of our professional, ethical

responsibility to give voice to the voiceless. I knew
the importance of a mindful pause before starting
operational meetings, to consciously pay homage to
a healing-caring connection. This reflection period
provides time for the nurse leader to recall their human
connection and interconnectedness. As promised, I
channeled the experience of Mr. and Mrs. C to fuel
the motivation to develop and implement the facility
PFCCM. The model was shared monthly at hospital and
nursing orientation meetings, and became integrated
into the fabric of the nursing community at our hospital.

For a year, Mr. C continued to visit me. He would
appear in the Nursing Administrative office, in formal
dress, and receive updates on the progression of the
PFCCM. I always made time for these unscheduled
visits, politely excusing myself from meetings, in order
to enjoy our healing conversations. I observed him move
through the stages of grief throughout the year as I
learned more about Mrs. C and their life journey as
husband and wife. During his last visit he shared with
me his decision to move away from the area to be
closer to family.

His final visit was bittersweet as I came to realize the
beautiful, transpersonal caring relationship that had
unfolded throughout the year. I had seen his gentle soul
progress through stages of grief, as he regained his voice

and new sense of self, without his beloved wife at his side.

The caring relationship transformed my spirit as a nurse and CNO. I gained clarity of purpose as I modeled Caritas practices, while leading the nursing community and proudly integrated a PFCCM... fueled with the inner light and spirit of Mr. and Mrs. C.

A Hairy Situation

Elin Høyvik Assistant Professor, RN, MSc
Haugesund, Norway

I used to work as a patrol nurse. During a reform, we had to scrutinize every single aspect of the help we provided in the patients' homes. We were told to remove every single activity that was considered unnecessary, in order to obtain a more sustainable health care. One of the tasks on our daily schedule is to put rollers in a woman's hair if they had curls. The process of rolling a woman's hair is time-consuming, and was not viewed as necessary by our leaders in the process of removing obsolete procedures.

This discussion caused quite a debate amongst the nurses, and many nurses were divided in this matter. Personally, I valued the time spent rolling the patients' hair. Even though I have other tasks in their homes, to care for a person's hair gives time and presence for deeper conversations. We often would talk about matters that are more personal to the patient as things slowed down, and my attention became more sharpened. One woman shared a very romantic story about how she and her husband first met. Sharing interpersonal moments like this allows us to form a closer relationship, as we are not just nurse and patient, but two people sharing a moment that brought us closer together.

One of Watson`s ten caritive factors explains why nursing practice as described above is necessary, as it creates a space to naturally form human connections. To roll someone's hair could be considered a trivial act without substance, but this process allows for us nurses to be attentive towards the patient. Taking care of the hair shows the patient that she is important to me, and that I am here for her.

The Novice And The Grieving Widow

Elin Høyvik Assistant Professor, RN, MSc
Haugesund, Norway

As a newly educated nurse, many of the regular staff at the nursing home were on holiday during a summer in the late 1990s. One day there were many substitutes on the ward, many of them new to the caring profession. This put me in a position of a lot of responsibility, in which I was not fully prepared for at the time. One of the assistants informed me that a resident had passed away. This sent me into a state of panic, as it became apparent how little I knew of procedures and ways to approach deaths at the nursing home. As I franticly searched folder after folder for guidelines, the resident's widow arrived in the hallway. This married couple was very familiar to me, as I had visited their home several times as a patrol nurse. They were both a delight, and the nursing staff enjoyed time with them, as they would laugh and tease us during these visits.

When the woman saw me coming out of the office she cried, "There you are," as she threw her arms around me and held tight. I felt clueless and did not know what to say or do. The woman did not let go of me, and that told me that I needed to be present. I asked her if she wanted to go into the room where her husband lay, and she agreed. She held my hand tightly as we walked together into the room to say goodbye to her husband. With one hand holding mine, she stroked the face of her husband, as she thanked him for the many wonderful years they shared together. Her grief became mine, and I could envision the two of them sharing a lifetime of happiness together. We were connected not just by holding hands, but also on a much deeper level.

This moment felt so much bigger and more powerful than either of us could comprehend. Although I felt insecure about how to take care of this woman in her mourning, I knew that she welcomed my presence. I felt gratitude towards the widow because she *chose me* to accompany her during what might have been the most difficult time in her life.

As a young and unexperienced nurse, I lacked both theoretical and practical knowledge to address this situation. However, we shared something sacred beyond words. This encounter had an immense impact on me, and it taught me that caring situations take many forms. Nursing schools do not teach us how to handle difficult situations specifically, but meeting someone in authenticity allows the moment to evolve in an organic matter. Twenty years following this incident, getting to know Watson`s theory of Human Caring made me think of this moment I shared with the grieving widow.

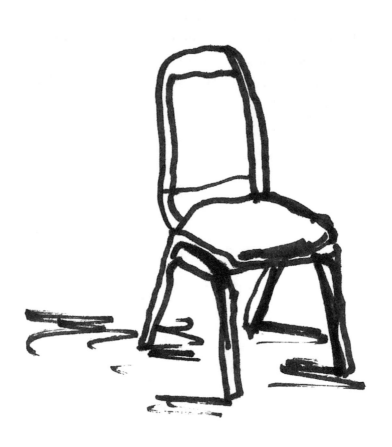

Caritas Process 5

Allowing for expression of positive and negative feelings — authentically listening to another person's story.

The Trauma Behind The Anger

Holly Clanton BSN, RN, CCRN, CHPN

Menomonee Falls, Wisconsin, USA

Throughout my 27 year career as a nurse, I have cared for many patients that are termed "difficult." What I have learned is that if I can identify the reason behind the emotion I can typically form a better working relationship with them. Some patients act out in fear, others in anger, some in distrust or confusion. I recently had an experience with such a patient. To me hearing his story on admission was sad. He had experienced homelessness and had multiple mental health diagnoses. His admitting diagnosis to our hospice/palliative care unit was end stage cancer and he was being admitted for end of life stay.

Some years back he had chosen a POA (Power of Attorney) that worked at the hospital in a different area. This woman had befriended him along his many years in our system and she conveyed that he truly had no family members interested in maintaining a relationship with him.

He arrived on our unit angry and bitter, which continued throughout his stay. He was resistant to every attempt made to help him, whether it was to help with his pain or ADLs (Activities of Daily Living). He would yell, swear, make vulgar statements, throw things, and was a danger to himself and others. He had a history of leaving the hospital AMA (Againgst Medical Advice). Now however, his disease was progressing to the point he was physically unable to care for himself. Psychology staff offered suggestions and boundaries were set which he continuously pushed beyond their limits.

The staff on our unit was exhausted in attempting to provide care to this patient who made it very clear he was not appreciative of our efforts. Into the second week of this continuous abusive behavior, I was working the night shift and after tending to the duties of my other patients, I took the time to enter his room and sat down. He yelled, "What the fuck are you doing sitting in my room? Get the fuck out! It's not like any of you bitches care anyways." I had chosen to sit near the door a safe distance away from him so he could not reach me physically (he was too weak to get out of bed). All potential objects that he could have thrown were no longer allowed within his reach. I remained seated and allowed him to yell. When he took a second to catch his breath, I calmly asked him, "Why are you so angry?" I sat and waited for his response. Again he went off yelling profanities and accusing us of "not giving two shits about him or anyone else." I sat and allowed him to vent. I then calmly said again, "I am here, and I want to know why are you so angry?" He then looked me straight in the face, which was unusual for him because normally he would scream and yell, avoiding your gaze unless he was throwing something. (I knew he had nothing to throw so I felt safe). "Do you really want to know why I am so angry?" he asked. "Yes. I am here to listen, tell me your story" I answered. He said, "Well, if you really want to fucking know here's why I am so angry: When I was in Vietnam I was in a platoon. This kid had just been sent to join us. He was 18 or 19 years old. One minute he was in front of me, and the next minute I saw his fucking head splattered all over the place. He was just a kid. He had a life to live. That's why I'm fucking angry and this place doesn't give a shit about that kid, me, or anyone else."

We both sat silent for a minute or two. I noticed his hands were shaking as he told the story and continued now. His breathing was deep as he tried to hold back his emotions. I looked him in the face and said slowly and purposefully, "Thank you for sharing your story. I am sorry for what you experienced and I am sorry for the boy's death and those of so many others during Vietnam.

I am here because I do care. We can't change those horrific experiences. But we can listen and we can help you if you let us."

I sat there for a few more minutes and he refused to look at me. I left the room without saying any more and closed his door as he had always preferred. Throughout that evening and the following days he was calmer. His behavior was no longer abusive towards staff, it was more indifferent. He died within a week of sharing his story with me. Based on the change in his behavior, I believe I may have been one of a few or maybe the only person he shared this tragedy with. I believe that by authentically listening and allowing safe place to share his story without judgment, he was able to achieve a more peaceful death.

The Heart-shaped Bloodstain

Joycelyn Cudjoe PhD, RN
Herndon, Virginia, USA

The first time I met my patient, I took care of him for just three hours. His nurse had to leave the unit, so I stepped in to take care of him while she was away. I went into my patient's room around 4pm to introduce myself. Our interaction was very brief. Prior to leaving the hospital that evening (it was my last shift for the week), I went to his room to say goodbye. He asked me if I would be his nurse the following week if he was not discharged. I agreed. I was not surprised when I returned to work five days later to see his name on my patient assignment list and I smiled.

He was a 22-year-old man who was admitted to the hospital for a urinary tract infection and a left thigh abscess. He was paralyzed from the waist down as a result of a gunshot wound to his spine. After receiving report from the previous night shift nurse, I went into his room to introduce myself. I noticed he was covered from head to toe with 4 heavy blankets. I pulled the blanket down to see what was wrong. He immediately pulled the blankets over his head and yelled, "I don't want to talk right now! Leave me alone!" I agreed to give him a few minutes to regroup. The young man I had just interacted with was very different from the perky, lively young man I met the previous week. I knew something was wrong, and I needed to find out.

A few minutes later, I went back to his room. This time, his face was covered in tears. I closed his room curtains, pulled a chair next to his bed and sat. I did not ask any questions. I just sat. Amidst sobs, he said, "Nurse, I'm scared. I'm really scared."

"Scared of what?" I asked.

"The doctors said they may have to cut my legs off if this surgery does not go well."

Based on the report I received that morning, I knew he was scheduled for wound debridement and abscess drainage in the OR.

"The doctors said they are going to cut off my legs!" He screamed.

I explained what wound debridement meant and took time to answer all of his questions.

He quickly wiped his tears and began telling me about his childhood. His favorite childhood memory was singing hymns with his grandmother while she cooked lunch on Sundays. He also told me about the day he got shot. While we were talking, the phlebotomist came in to draw blood samples. During the procedure, a drop of blood fell onto his blanket.

"Hey, take a look at this," I said.

He carefully examined the blood stain. "Wow! It's shaped like a heart! This is crazy! What do you think it means?" he exclaimed. I smiled and said, "Why don't you tell me what it means to you?"

He closed his eyes and took in a deep breath. When he opened his eyes, they twinkled. With a broad, radiant smile, he said, "It's God speaking to me! I am alive today because God loves me. I was broken. My heart was broken. I was angry because I felt there was no way out of this mess I had gotten myself into. I grew up in the church. My grandma used to take me to church all the time, but I left the church and got on the wrong path. When I got shot, I was broken! Today, God has given me a sign. The heart-shaped blood is God's way of reminding me to trust in Him. God gave me this sign to remind me of the true meaning of love and life. The heart pumps blood to sustain human life. God wants me to know that he loves me. He can heal my broken heart."

Again, there was silence. This time, it was not an awkward silence. This silence signified hope. This silence signified trust. The small, heart-shaped bloodstain on the white hospital blanket, marked the beginning of a spiritual journey of peace, hope, and unwavering faith for a young man and his nurse.

Authentic Listening With Psychiatric Patients

Macy Powers BSN, RN
Greenville, North Carolina, USA

The fifth caritas is to promote and accept positive and negative feelings through authentic listening. This is something that as a pediatric nurse I have to use on a daily basis. Because I work on a pediatric intermediate floor, we accept all patients including psych patients. I had a 14-year-old patient that was admitted for an intentional overdose. She had taken forty plus pills in an attempt to take her own life. This was her second suicide attempt, and she previously has been in inpatient psych three times. When I admitted her, she was very quiet and kept to herself. She would not answer any of my questions or even make eye contact with me. Once she was settled into her room and her family left, I went in to try to have a conversation with her. Instead of asking her questions about why she took the pills or about her depression, I asked her about her personal life. I asked her what she liked to do in her spare time, what she wanted to do when she was older, etc. We talked for almost an hour and by the end of the conversation she even laughed a few times. She explained to me that I was the first person to listen to her and not look at her for the situation she was in. Authentic listening is so important in nursing because these patients often don't have someone to listen to them. As a nurse I always try to remember this, especially with my teenage patients.

Finding Comfort in the Process

Kelli Stangel RN, BSN, CHPN
Spokane, Washington, USA

I chose to reflect on Caritas Process 5, in realizing I need more work in this arena. I need a bit more 'cloud grasping' in my day to day, as I often find myself, 'holding onto' offenses, or trying to come up with a solution to someone's problems — while they are still mid-story. It is quite challenging for me to stay totally present, in the moment and engaged, as I am more tempted to offer to fix whatever issue they are sharing. I suppose I'm not a fan of the process. I'm more a fan of the ending and the quicker I can get to the ending the better, which I acknowledge is not the best answer for those I work with who are needing to work through issues, rather than be spoon-fed an answer. Decreasing the number of repetitive issues based on processing the current one (and thereby becoming invested in the solution) should be the goal here, versus, being told: "Here's what I'm going to do about it for you."

I manage a staff of twelve: eleven females, one male. I struggle to keep my mind open and my mouth shut when presented with one more encounter of the "he said/she said" scenario. I have come to realize that what makes sense to me in my life does not always translate to others, nor is it helpful to hand them a quick fix. Patience is not my strength. Every time a staff person has an issue and I give them a solution to ease my negative feelings, I cripple them. I rob them of sitting in the discomfort which acts as motivation to find an answer. I realize that any shortcut I take or make for them simply puts off the inevitable, for as long as they are spoon-fed, they have a much lower chance of actually owning the problem, pondering possible solutions, and experiencing the process it took to resolve it, walking away with a new history of problem solving.

I have plenty of examples when I have gotten in my own way as well as the staff's, putting in twice the work, twice the number of meetings and emails — all because I was slow to realize that I am not here to dole out answers or take away another's discomfort as they navigate toward a solution. Nor should I try to alleviate my own uneasiness as that feeling becomes a motivating factor for change, and I need to allow it its own space in the room. As I become more comfortable with being uncomfortable, the staff will be empowered to experience the process of conflict management and be more apt to accept/own the outcome, being part of/invested in it.

As a nurse I always thought I was here to relieve suffering, even minor discomforts. As growth and learning take place, I realize I have been shortchanging myself and the staff, often missing the opportunity to experience and thus comprehend the true meaning of lovingkindness, selflessness, and teamwork.

The Story of Ruth

Carole Bergin RN, CHTP
Arlington, Virginia, USA

I have known this patient for over a decade. She is a patient with multiple complicated medical problems. Her life situation is not optimal, neither in her personal life nor her work situation.

I first met her as a pre-surgical patient. Ruth is a "frequent flyer" at the hospital. Everyone knows her. She calls us her family. Ruth is great at asking for help and stating her needs clearly which is such a gift. During her interview with me, I listened to her concerns about being MRSA positive and her desire to have that label removed prior to her surgery. I heard her, and ensured that the process was achieved for her. She had everything imaginable wrong with her including many allergies and complications from surgeries gone awry. I listened to each story. She came to trust me and to feel that she was heard and cared for.

I have seen her monthly for years, even if it was just passing her by in the lab waiting room. In the last several years I have seen her in the infusion center receiving treatment more frequently, at least once or twice a month. I provide her Healing Touch (HT) with the goal of bringing her positive, healing energy. She absorbs HT with much gratitude and she notices a percentage of change in her ailments and how she feels emotionally as a whole. Part of Healing Touch is connection between two people. I am someone she can vent her frustrations to, and can listen with sincerity. I try to place a positive spin on her failing body by affirming her strengths. I listen to her disappointment with her family and work relationships. I revel with her in her happy moments. She says our connection and Healing Touch is her lifeline.

I am personally inspired by her ability to survive — even thrive — with all her problems. After all these years, she has given *me* as much as I have supported her. I find her awesome... a pillar of a woman. It is funny how this symbiotic relationship has been good for both of us.

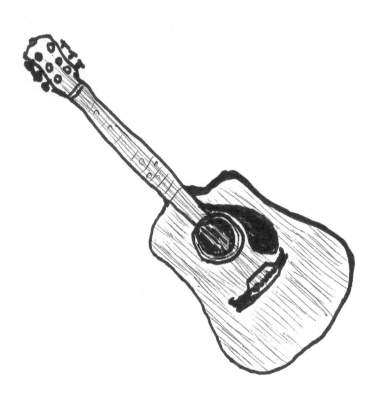

Caritas Process 6

Creatively problem-solving, 'solution-seeking' through caring process; full use of self and artistry of caring-healing practices via use of all ways of knowing/being/doing/becoming.

A Knock At The Door

Mary Tolliver BSN, RNC-OB
Women's Health Navigator
Leesburg, Virginia, USA

A letter of desperation was written to one of our OBGYNs (Obstetrical & Gynecological Doctor) by a patient who was experiencing unpredictable menstrual flow and pain that would last ten to fourteen days at a time and was affecting her quality of life and mental health. She reported feeling depressed and having suicidal thoughts prior to her periods; something she said she had never experienced in her life. This young woman described how she felt like she was, "in the middle of the ocean, drowning and there is no land in sight. It had been hours upon days trying to stay afloat and I just want to give up and let go." She went on to write that she had never been or felt so hopeless in her life. These feelings were overwhelming and she felt so helpless that she did not want to be alive. These thoughts and feelings were affecting her quality of life and everything she did.

In the letter she pleaded for help, stating she did not know what else to do.

The OBGYN forwarded his letter to me. Immediately upon reading it, I felt a sense of urgency for this woman's safety due to her thoughts of self harm. The psychiatric liaison was consulted for advice on how to manage this outpatient's care. I called the young woman's home and cell phones with no response. I left a voice message informing her that her doctor asked me to follow up with her and requested a return call. I called her job; she had called in sick. I called the local police and requested a wellness check. As my anxiety began to soar, the patient returned my call. I introduced myself as the Women's Health Navigator, and informed her that her doctor was very concerned about her and had shared her letter with me. I listened empathically as she explained how desperate and hopeless she was feeling. I thanked her for sharing her most intimate thoughts and feelings. I told her how concerned I was for her safety and wellbeing and asked her to come into the emergency department for an evaluation and to receive mental health resources. She was hesitant, but after speaking with me for some time, she agreed to come to the emergency department as long as I would meet her there.

I went to the emergency department and waited for her to arrive. After some time, with concern, I called the patient to see where she was. She told me that she had decided to go to the emergency department closer to her home, and asked if I could meet her there. I notified my supervisor of the change in plans and without hesitation, my supervisor agreed. On my way to meet her, the patient called and explained her sister in-law had told her that the hospital is for 'severe problems,' and that if she went there, they will put her 'in the looney house.' The patient got scared and decided to go home and said she would not come back. I asked the patient for her address, notified my supervisor, and headed to her home. I knocked on her door.

A beautiful young woman greeted me with tear filled eyes and a big grateful hug.

With compassion and empathy, I spoke with the patient for a few minutes before her boyfriend arrived. After speaking with them both, and expressing my concern for her safety, the patient agreed to go back to the emergency room for a wellness check. En route, I notified my supervisor and the Emergency Department team leader that I was escorting the patient and her boyfriend to the department for suicidal ideation. I left once the patient felt comfortable with the care she was receiving. The patient was assessed and later discharged home with resources for community mental health services. This patient was pleading for help and she was beyond grateful to receive it.

Since the incident the patient has been going to counseling.

A Birth Navigator Program Exemplar

Cindy Andrejasich MSN, RNC, NE-BC
Purcellville, Virginia, USA

In October of 2009, we officially launched our Birth Navigator program.

For years, we have offered personalized consultations with a labor & delivery nurse to answer questions, address concerns, and help the mother achieve the birth experience that she is hoping for. Previously however, this has always been carried out within an informal structure.

The Birth Navigator program formalized this process, giving each family a contact person to advise and advocate for them throughout their pregnancy and delivery.

One such collaboration between myself and a family, was a couple with unique concerns. It was a same-sex couple in a committed relationship who had endured extended challenges with infertility, and with no positive result as yet, to show for their emotional and financial investment.

Facing their last possible cycle of in-vitro fertilization due to financial constraints, the couple made the rather courageous decision for both of them to attempt implantation, in order to maximize their chance of finally achieving a pregnancy. This was accomplished by having eggs harvested by one of the potential moms, but for each half of the eggs to be fertilized by one of two different donors. This decision was made because there had been a previous issue with embryonic quality, directly related to the sperm donor.

Imagine the surprise of these hopeful mothers when not one, but both of these implantations resulted in healthy pregnancies! This couple presented to me several months before delivery with their desire to proactively manage their labor and delivery processes. There were many variables and concerns to consider, since their estimated date of delivery was obviously the same for each of them.

The first meeting was spent discussing and exploring all possible logistical scenarios, as well as establishing a relationship of comfort and trust. It was of utmost importance that this couple be made to feel that they were in a place of acceptance and support, and that they understood how privileged we felt to be able to assist them with this wonderful, albeit unique experience. We mapped out (as best we could) every possible algorithm, including the most challenging: the simultaneous labour of both moms.

Throughout the subsequent weeks, I kept in contact with the couple, answering questions and offering encouragement. Other members of the healthcare team were included in the process in order to maintain a multidisciplinary approach, and to increase the couple's level of comfort with our staff. Happily, our two mothers ended up going into labor six days apart from each other, which gave each mom the opportunity to have her unique birth experience with the support of her partner, along with the nursing staff. With the birth of the second child, we made arrangement for the entire family to "room-in" together in our Post-partum unit, and everyone couldn't have been happier.

It was such a joy to walk in for rounds in the morning, and see both moms happily breastfeeding their beautiful babies within the comfort and support of our staff. This family left us feeling grateful, and we were forever changed by meeting this family 'where they were', and doing whatever we could to give them the experience that they deserved.

The Power
of Music

Raymond Leone MMT, MT-BC
Leesburg, Virginia, USA

In the hospital where I work as a music therapist, I was recently called to work by a young gentleman and his wife in the oncology unit. She had requested a visit after overhearing me provide music therapy in another room. Having both been born and raised in South America, they both speak some English but not a lot, and had been living in the US for the past few years. He was very ill. He had an advanced stage of cancer and was declining rapidly. At this point the goals of care are 'comfort' (although he unfortunately didn't look very comfortable). He was in a great deal of pain and had also lost his ability to swallow. He really couldn't speak much and was very frail. When I walked into the room, he looked at me and his eyes said it all — he was moving towards transitioning and seemingly dealing with both physical and emotional distress. She was by his side and looked... lost. They were both in their early thirties.

She smiled and offered her hand, and thanked me for coming. There was certainly a language barrier between us but, I have music, so I sat and brought some music into their current world. I was thinking 'comfort' and imagining what they were both going through as I played, improvising on the guitar.

During these situations, I work to provide a soundscape that is both soothing and reflective. I was trying to 'hold' them both, together... with the music. He focused on the guitar as I played; perhaps having something to fixate on, taking his focus away from everything else. She held his hand and just looked at him.

After about 20 minutes or so, with a natural ebb in the music, he gave me a faint smile and a very slight 'thumbs up.' When she saw that, she was suddenly beaming and looked at me and softly said, "Thank you." "What is your favorite music? I asked her, Is there anything you can tell me about his favorite music?" She paused, perhaps trying to translate what she wanted to say in her head, then sheepishly said, "We like Hotel California," with almost an embarrassed little laugh. I said, "Oh, okay. Can I play it for you?" She looked at him and then said, "Please... we met in California." And now trying to hold back tears, "It's... our song."

During the song, they held hands and at times looked

like teens at a high school dance and other times, as
though fear and uncertainty was going to take over.
But… it was a beautiful moment. A beautiful and
peaceful moment that was created by the power of a
meaningful song. I can't imagine there were too many
"beautiful moments" for them in recent days or whatever
days were left to come. But in this moment — smiles…
love… connection… music.

It feels strange to say I feel lucky I got to share this
moment with them — in a hospital room in an oncology
unit at the very near end — but I do. I was lucky to have
been able to facilitate a moment for them that was so
needed. I was lucky to see something that was not pain
nor fear in their eyes for a moment. Sure, it was only a
song. One song and just a moment. At this point in the
game, there really isn't anything else that can be given
during this kind of moment… other than music. What
else could bring a smile and some comfort (yes, comfort)
at this point? When there is nothing left, we still have
music… meaningful music. The healing power of music.

From Cruise to Caring Practice

Zach Wotherspoon DNP, APRN, FNP-BC,
RN, CEN, CPEN
Stafford, Virginia, USA

As a leader in an acute care facility, I enjoy touching the lives of the care team equally as much as impacting the lives of those we are privileged to serve. I hired an experienced nurse onto our unit who demonstrated the qualities we all look for in each other: accountability, kindness, and integrity. Interested in pursuing his Doctor of Nursing Practice degree with a concentration as a Family Nurse Practitioner, I was impressed by this person's drive to achieve his goals.

One Sunday I received a call from our charge nurse to report this nurse had called out for his shift that night as well as his next shift scheduled for Tuesday due to feeling ill. It is somewhat peculiar to receive a phone call calling out for numerous shifts, especially when they are not concurrent, due to an illness. I attempted to contact the team member on Wednesday to check on him to see how he was progressing. I was not able to reach him and tried again to reach him via phone on Thursday. Unable to reach him, I left a message stating that I hoped he was feeling better and also inquiring about his upcoming shift on that Saturday. The nurse called me back on Friday and informed me that he was not going to be in on Saturday either; he did not sound ill on the phone and I began to have a feeling there was an underlying issue that was not being mentioned.

The following week, the nurse returned to work and came into my office and closed the door. After well wishes he explained to me that he was not unwell the prior week and instead was on a cruise with his family that his mother had gifted to them. Without giving me an opportunity to speak, he accepted his fate of a final written warning or termination, claiming that spending that time and making memories with his aging mother was worth any degree of accountability he was to face. He continued with remorse for leaving his co-workers less-staffed, but continued to be accepting of any fate that lie ahead.

As a leader, one must acknowledge their feelings of frustration and disappointment; more importantly, a leader must also evaluate the larger picture and understand how such circumstances can develop and sustain loving, trusting-caring relationships. Knowing this nurse was interested in pursuing graduate studies, but lacking confidence to embark on the journey, I made a proposal. First, I thanked him for his honesty in acknowledging the hardship that he placed on his peers. I then inquired about his graduate application for which he denied completing.

Choosing to hold him accountable in a positive, hopeful, and compassionate manner; I asked that he please submit to me confirmation of a submitted graduate application by the end of the following week. During the course of that week and a half, I assisted him by reviewing his resume and essays, and coached him through the application process. It was clear to me that this man was remorseful and took responsibility for his actions, so what was progressive discipline truly likely to achieve?

Two years later, this nurse continues to be one of the highest performers I have worked with and has transitioned into a leadership role whereby he is able to support and empower others. Furthermore, this nurse was accepted into the DNP-FNP program he applied to and started his FNP clinical rotations in May 2020. Accepting this person's feelings through authentically listening to his story, accepting his needs and motivations, and using compassion as a driver for accountability both retained this high-performer and assisted with motivating him to pursue his personal and professional goals.

Watching Baseball with a Beer in Hand

Irene Flores MSN, RN, ONC

Fairfax, Virginia, USA

Being an oncology nurse is not all about delivering sad news, giving chemo or controlling pain. We develop relationships, getting to know our patients and what brings joy to their lives. This past fall as baseball season was coming to an end, the Washington National were going to the World Series. Our hospital is just miles away from the nation's capital.

How does a nurse cheer up Nationals fans that are in a hospital bed receiving or recovering from chemotherapy? Creativity & coordination of care, a phone call to the oncologist to get an order for non-alcoholic beer, chips, hotdogs and chicken wings.

As the nursing leader on the unit, I know which patients are baseball fans, as we had talked about our team during my rounding. I left work early, ran over to the grocery store, bought all the supplies, and came back to the hospital. My staff looked at me as if I had lost my mind. They had never seen a nursing leader do such a thing.

Our Nationals fans had the best World Series game they could have asked for, their team won. The next day so many people stopped by my office to thank me, and a couple of patients said, "There is nothing like watching baseball with a beer in hand."

A Beautiful Wedding

Margaret Stewart BA, BSN, RN, PCCN

Aldie, Virginia, USA

I was a week or so off of orientation as a new grad
RN. This was my first job since graduating with my
second Degree: BSN. I had done a lot of other odd jobs
before arriving at this one — including making wedding
dresses! One day at work, we received a patient with end-
stage cancer. She was not our usual diagnosis, because
we usually take care of people after cardiothoracic
surgery. But whatever the cause — fate or bed availability
— she ended up with us. Her disease was so progressive
that she only had a very short time to live. In light of
this, she decided to marry her longterm partner as soon
as she could. She wasn't going to be able to leave the
hospital, so we decided to put on a wedding for them!
My manager ordered flowers and a cake and organized
the chaplain... But what would the bride wear?

Why, a Grecian-inspired, softly draping and gathered
dress made out of bedsheets, pins, and silk tape, of

course! Miss S., as I'll call her, cried when I turned her around to look in the mirror. She said she felt beautiful. All those folds of stiff cotton had been transformed into something that made her smile, and concealed, "all the bits that needed concealing," in her words.

We gussied her up, popped her in a wheelchair, and rolled her downstairs. The couple took pictures in our courtyard, kissing and crying, and looking as beautiful and happy as every bride and groom should.

I was honored to care for this patient in a way that was seemingly completely unrelated to the nursing care I had learned in school. It was an honor to be able to offer Miss S. my artistic expression and expertise, and add to her life with creativity and imagination. It may not have been, strictly speaking, nursing care, but we were able to infuse her life with spontaneity, and with joy, in her last few days. That was the most beautiful dress I've ever made, and will ever make. I'll never forget her, and the gift that it was to offer my gifts to her.

Caritas Process 7

Engaging in transpersonal teaching and learning within context of caring relationship; staying within other's frame of reference — shift toward coaching model for expanded health/wellness.

Authentic Caring Leadership: "I couldn't until I did."

Pat McClendon RN, DNP, Caritas Coach
Temecula, California, USA

As a Chief Nursing Officer (CNO), I had reached a point where I knew I needed to find incremental ways to lead authentic caring in a direct and personal way. For years I had longed to apply caring science in my everyday leadership practice. I believed deeply in the reciprocal healing benefits of authentic caring for patients and nurses. Somehow I needed to give voice to that belief and engage nurses around it.

But I was stuck, always waiting for the right time, waiting for conflicting demands to resolve, or waiting to roll out a caring science program. Now I realize that

I was really waiting for me to be personally ready. At that moment I accepted that even though as a CNO I may not know how to directly help nurses expand their authentic caring awareness and skills, I could at least start talking more intentionally about authentic caring. I began with my nursing leadership team, then I started asking nurses about their authentic caring experiences, thoughts and feelings in classes, committee meetings, nursing forums and when rounding.

To my shock and surprise, several nurses opened up thoughtfully and authentically and with gratitude — Even when they were busy! Granted, I saw bewilderment come across other nurses' faces when they heard my question — as if they hadn't thought about their deep authentic caring feelings in a long time. And some nurses struggled to even consider this as an option in their work. But enough nurses engaged in meaningful ways. And if they couldn't share their stories and thoughts when I came around, they would find me on other days. The lesson learned was that nurses can and want to talk about their authentic caring experiences, even when they are busy.

I was launched. Connecting with nurses in meaningful ways motivated me to engage more with nurses, to round more, to speak more about caring across all work settings, and to think more about caring. I discovered that I did have time for leading authentic caring. And I discovered that nurses — especially young nurses — were hungry for these conversations.

Authentic caring is about momentary human connections that can have lasting effects. It's more about each nurse's level of awareness than it is about having time. That's why each nurse has to discover this individually. Leaders, being there to affirm nurses' incremental discoveries, expands our individual and collective caring consciousness. As nurses expand their consciousness along with their ability to authentically engage with patients around the demands of their work, nurse leaders can be there to add caring language to the experiences and to say, "Wow!"

My basic conversations with nurses about their caring practices and experiences evolved into caring engagement conversations. My self-doubt dissolved, as I trusted the process. We don't have to be gurus to lead authentic caring cultivation; we have our own experiences and evolving caring consciousness to share. "Show your humanity and no one will turn away" (Doty, 2017).

Caring engagement conversations is an organic nurse leader practice which centers around momentary and episodic exchanges between a nurse and a leader. They are do-able by any nurse leader, anywhere, in between seeing patients and other meetings. Cultivation of caring consciousness is an individual, personal discovery process. Nurse leaders being present to witness the nurse's process, however briefly, helps make it real and gives it meaning for each nurse. Caring engagement conversations can be used in conjunction with other caring initiatives or as a stand-alone practice (McClendon, 2019). Conversations about caring have always been important, but often have been squeezed out by other demands. There is nothing new here. These conversations thread through Nursing's history since Nightingale and are just as relevant today.

Nurse leaders are wedged between two major forces — medicine and business — dulling one's nursing sensibilities, philosophically and practically. Caring easily morphs into structures and measures, and loses authenticity. I was one of many well-intentioned nurse leaders who could not find a do-able way to personally impact nurses and caring practice until I did. How nurse leaders activate their authentic caring leader selves takes many paths.

It was my personal journey into wellness consciousness that awakened me — fueled by self-help, self-care and inner work. There is a wellness renaissance happening all around us evident in the groundswell of wellness programs in all walks of life that are informing our patients. Wellness programs and lifestyle research abound with evidence that authentic human connections heal suffering.

Nursing is ever evolving. Nursing's history has paralleled the evolution of the human experience and society's health, healing and caring needs within the consciousness of the time. Currently, society's needs reflect wellness consciousness — authenticity and human connectedness. Patients are not only seeking medical care in their healthcare encounters, they are seeking authentic human connections. And it is nurses to whom they are turning for that connection, as seen in patient experience metrics. Watson once wrote, "The change will come when nursing and nurses are directly aligned with the people they serve" (Watson, 1999, 46). That time is here. Nurses caring consciousness cultivation is as critical as nurses clinical mastery for the well-being of patients, nurses, organizational cultures, and society.

Nursing leadership's unique challenge is to embolden a nurse's covenant with society within the magnitude and scope of nursing and caring science. Only nurse leaders can make authentic caring a visible, active, and conscious part of our work environments. How nurse leaders lead caring, impacts how caring is recognized, understood, and valued by all within the healthcare industry. Conversations about caring weave meaning and purpose into a nurse's work, relationships, caring consciousness, and environments — helping us to thrive in nursing every day. This is our nurse leader legacy.

References

Doty JR. (October 26.2017). 'Alphabet of the heart.' Keynote: 23rd International Caritas Consortium. Watson Caring Science Institute & Stanford Health Care.

McClendon P. (2019). *Getting real about caring.* Bloomington, IN: AuthorHouse.

Watson J. (1999). *Postmodern nursing and beyond.* Edinburgh, Scotland: Churchill-Livingstone.

Honor Walk

Donna Thomas MSN, RN, Clinical Nurse Educator
Alexandria, Virginia, USA

It was a particularly quiet day in the ICU; as quiet
as it can be for an ICU. Our program director showed
up unannounced to observe participants for a research
project. He wanted to observe all of our ventilated
patients. That day there was only one: a forty-six-year-
old mom that had experienced a seizure, anoxic brain
injury, and subsequent brain death. Her family had
graciously decided to donate her organs. A new nurse
and her preceptor cared for her and discussed the
protocols. This was the new nurse's first experience with
a patient death.

The patient was not a candidate for the research
project. However, instead of packing up and heading
back to his office, our program director stayed and
suggested that we do an "Honor Walk" for this
patient. As a small ICU we had no experience with
this. He supported the unit and administration as they
went through the proper procedures. Staff from all
departments showed up and lined the hallways of her
ICU room to the elevator, and from the elevator to the

operating room where she was wheeled in for her final surgery. As they wheeled her into the operating room, the preceptor noticed the patient's brother standing among the staff. He was saluting his sister, a veteran. The family remained with her in the operating room as she was terminally extubated, and they each were able to say their final goodbyes.

While an incredibly sad outcome for the patient and her family, we were all uplifted by the way we "showed up" as a team to honor her, both for her life and for her gift to others. The new nurse remarked how humbling this experience had been for her. She saw the beauty in this gesture and witnessed how it helped the family cope with their grief of losing her — knowing that a part of her would go on to help others live.

The freedom to care for our patients as human beings and thanking them for their sacrifice, was very powerful for our unit. We were reminded to slow down and remember that the purpose of our work is to serve our patients while respecting their humanity and dignity. This was a day none of us on the unit will ever forget.

Caring Hearts

Natalie Hardee BSN, RN

Greenville, North Carolina, USA

Caritas Process 7 means to be fully present and aware in certain situations of what creates hope and faith in other individuals. As nurses I believe that we see this very often in our line of work whether we watch this happening to others or are the ones embodying this Caritas. I can think of many times that I have witnessed or been the health care professional going above and beyond for patients and creating a hopeful environment while in the hospital. However one situation in particular involving a physician sticks out to me the most.

We had a patient that was from a foreign country visiting family in the United States when she became ill and needed to be admitted to the hospital for a cardiac workup. This woman did not speak English and her family could not be at the hospital often due to their jobs. We utilized the MARTTI Cart as often as possible, but this was not creating a hopeful or spiritual environment for her. One of our physicians found out that this woman was from the same country as herself.

She began to visit the patient multiple times

throughout the day to speak with the patient, and discuss her medical plan, as well as just having conversations that most of the staff were unable to participate in. Our physician noticed that the patient was not eating as well as she needed to be, and so the physician cooked an authentic meal from their culture and brought it to her, which she devoured. All of the staff noticed a change in the patient as she became more eager to participate in physical therapy, and was generally more open to our care. The patient was eventually discharged to a rehab facility closer to her family.

To this day I believe that our physician being present with this patient and creating hope, helped her to more positively recover from her cardiac event.

A New Favorite Nursing Course

Joy Shepard PhD, RN-BC, CNE, CDP

Greenville, North Carolina, USA

The emphasis within Caritas Process 7, is on effective teaching and learning. Genuine teaching is transpersonal, powerfully affecting both parties within the teaching encounter. Thus, the relationship has the potential of continuing well past the teaching occasion, in exerting a lasting effect upon the life and behavior of participants (Sitzman & Watson, 2014; Watson, 2008). I always tell my students at the beginning of the semester that classroom learning is a two-way street; that I learn just as much from them as they do from me. I don't want to merely be the, "sage on the stage" as I teach in the classroom setting, but rather the, "guide on the side," facilitating their learning by actively engaging them in the learning process. I want to create a rich and diverse learning environment, where learning is celebrated and a lifelong love for learning engendered.

Combs, Avila, and Purkey (1971), examined the

factors that influence a teacher's effectiveness, to help determine what creates teaching effectiveness. They concluded that while subject-matter knowledge, methodological expertise, and theoretical perspective are necessary for effective teaching, the factors that are of paramount importance in distinguishing effective and ineffective teachers are the attitudinal, affective, and perceptual values — in other words, the beliefs that teachers hold concerning one's subject, others, oneself (self-concept), the purposes of helping, and beliefs about approaches to one's particular task. "The interchange between a teacher and (learners) will be different every moment, and the teacher must be prepared to react to each (learner) in terms of the unique question, idea, problem, and concern that he is expressing at that particular instant" (Combs et al., 1971, p. 5). According to their seminal research, effective teachers possess the following attributes or beliefs: learner oriented; focused on learners; the belief that learners are able to solve their own problems if given the proper tools to do so; the belief that learners are worthy of dignity; identification with learners; positive self-image; not afraid to reveal "self" to learners; have a "freeing" approach (solution-focused versus problem-focused); and focus on larger goals (search for authentic meaning, inner truth, and purpose and vision) (Combs et al., 1971).

The sacredness of each and everything we do brings to mind this famous quotation by Florence Nightingale: "Nursing is an art, and if it is to be an art, it requires as exclusive a devotion and as hard a preparation as any painter's or sculptor's work; for what is having to do with a dead canvas or cold marble, compared to having to do with the living body — the temple of God's spirit? It is one of the fine arts; I would say the finest of the Fine Arts" (Florence Nightingale, 1860).

In terms of embodiment of the 7th and 8th Caritas processes, my colleague and I were given the honor and privilege of teaching a classroom course that in the past had generated much strife among the students, their parents, the faculty involved, and others. It had been labeled a "problem" course by some within our college, simply because of the way it had been taught over a continuing span of many years. The content material was outside of my scope of expertise (my area of expertise is gerontology and this course is pediatrics); however, the basic tenets of teaching-learning remain the same. In order to break this negative cycle, we had to start from "scratch" in totally redesigning the course. This involved much intense work and research, but it was worth it. We purposely made the course as "learner-friendly" as possible. We employed such tactics as making the course Powerpoints readily available to all the course learners on SlideShare, providing practice examinations with lots of instructor feedback, having pre-test as well as post-test reviews, and just making every student feel as if he or she was valued and important. We welcomed student input/feedback in the course, and were quick to respond to each and every one of their emails. All this meticulous planning and intentional caring paid off. For the first time in years, the students were pleased with the pediatrics course and feedback was overwhelmingly positive. The learning environment was welcoming, positive, caring, and healing. A little caring goes a long, long way.

References

Combs, A., Avila, D., & Purkey, W. (1971). *Helping relationships: Basic concepts for the helping professions.* Boston: Allyn & Bacon.

Watson, J. (2008). *Nursing: The philosophy and science of caring* (Rev. ed.) Boulder, CO: University Press of Colorado.

Serving a Vulnerable Population

Nina Reyes RN, BSN
Fairfax, Virginia, USA

I am blessed to work as a registered nurse where I can
provide service to others. In my RN Case Manager role,
I can practice humility, altruism, and empathy daily.
When I first took this job, I was told I could create it
to serve the population of patients with whom I work.
I was new to working in the community population of
vulnerable patients. Many of these patients are people
who have recently come to this country, do not have
insurance, and do not have access to education about
healthy lifestyles. I used to work in the hospital, where
the patients are literate, have health insurance, and are
less vulnerable. One of my tasks is to educate patients
about primary care health conditions; long term, if left
unmanaged, these conditions can cause major health

problems. I meet with patients to follow up about their blood pressure or glucose levels. Several of the patients I serve, do not understand their health conditions.

In the hospital, I had access to videos and other learning tools I could use to help educate the patients. In this community case management role, I do not have as many of these tools. Many of my patients only speak Spanish, have many barriers, and are illiterate. I had to think outside the box and simplify my teaching approach, in order to better serve them. Instead of overwhelming them with so much information at one time, I tailor each nurse visit to the comprehension of the individual patient. It is rewarding for me to see how grateful these patients are, to have this education.

Serving this population of patients is fulfilling. Each patient is thankful to have access to care, and have someone take the time to teach them about their condition. The most rewarding thing, is to see an improved outcome. I approach each visit with compassion and kindness; and practice with the mindset that this population is just unaware. It helps to humble me, to keep me present in each moment, to value my own health and blessings. In this role, I am able to coach my patients to help them improve their health. I have the opportunity to really know my patients and form meaningful relationships with them. Additionally,

I was able to practice Spanish and learn how to speak fluently. I have learned how to practice compassion and equanimity with myself, and others.

This experience has allowed me to recognize how fortunate I am to have these skills and be able to serve a vulnerable population.

The Waiting Room

Anna Biley Dip. N., M. Sc (Nursing), DCS.
Doctorate Caring Science, Faculty Associate WCSI
Dorchester, Dorset, England

The main quest of nursing research is to find out
what it means to be human at this moment in history
(Watson, 2018). In a safe space, Unitary Caring Science
invites creative modes of enquiry, probing new ways
of thinking, teaching and learning. Grounded in the
principle of caring transpersonal relationships, we
become a community of teachers/learners, co-creating
and deepening our understanding of caring, healing
and health. The experiences that connect us as human
beings, such as suffering, joy, grief, laughter, life and
death are at the core of creativity in art, poetry, music
and literature. Caring Science scholars have been at the
forefront of incorporating the arts into nurse education
and research and instrumental in making it a mainstream
approach to learning (Rosa, Horton-Deutsch & Watson,
2018).

In my own practice I often used a picture by the
English artist L.S. Lowry. The painting is entitled
Waiting Room, Ancoats Hospital, Salford (1964). Lowry

was famous for painting what he saw, scenes from everyday life in industrial, Northern England. His life. Although to many this may seem a grim subject, this is the place I was born and brought up. And so, I ask students, what do they see? What stories do the colours and shapes portray? What do they see in faces, eyes and clothing? Where is there gentleness and touch? What does the painting tell us about the people, their lives, health, happiness and dreams? Where is the humanity, care and dignity? What does the picture tell us about the healing environment?

Life is complex and in healthcare settings, even more so, but through exploration of art, a community of learners may share how experience and personal intuition help us see that there is always more going on than meets the eye. Being present, in the moment, in human-to-human relationship often reveals anxiety, stress, sadness, grief, trauma and fear. So often in healthcare, as in life, the focus is on problems and negative cycles of behaviour and relationships. In contrast, Caritas 7 encourages us to see beyond what we see, — the problem. Transpersonal teaching and learning spans and connects the caritas processes, to explore intention, presence, moments of caring and allows creative, kind actions and solutions to unfold that are grounded in listening, compassion and dignity.

References

Note from Editor:
You can view L.S Lowry
Waiting Room, Ancoats Hospital, Salford (1964) here:
art net.com/artists/ls-lowry/waiting-room-ancoats-hospital-
slaford-UNE31 FWEKXD-06GtGaGfow2
(addressed 18th July 2020).

Rosa, W., Horton-Deutsch, S. & Watson, J. (2018).
A handbook for caring science.
New York: Springer.

Watson, J. (2018). *Unitary caring science*. Louisville:
University Press of Colorado.

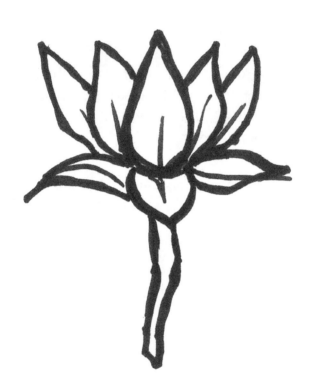

Caritas Process 8

Creating a healing environment at all levels; subtle environment for energetic authentic caring presence.

An Orientee in the ER

Irenious P. Suglo BSN, RN, CEN, CPEN
Bristow, Virginia, USA

While orienting a new graduate nurse in the ER, we were going to see a new patient that had just been brought back from triage. My orientee wanted to review a flag in the patient's chart before entering the room. Since flags can be for infectious diseases, I reviewed it with her. The flag turned out to be for violent conduct and described the patient's behavior as belligerent, accusatory, and cursing out healthcare workers. This flag painted the picture of an angry 85-year-old man with a history of being verbally abusive with hospital staff.

I looked at my orientee and told her to erase everything we had just read from her mind, and I instructed her that I did not want her to remember any of that or think about it while we were in the patient's room. With shock on her face, she asked me, "Why?" I informed her that I don't particularly appreciate introducing myself to patients with any preconceived judgment because we do not know what kind of emotional state either the patient or the practitioner who flagged his chart, was in during this incident. It is always a good idea to approach someone with a fresh mind that is void of any judgment, because people can feel it when you are suspicious or worried that they may be abusive to you. Then they will be guarded, and you will not get the whole story and may walk away with confirmation that "Yup, he or she is definitely a curmudgeon."

When we entered the room and introduced ourselves, the first thing the patient said to us was, "I don't even know why I'm here because y'all are all the same, and no one cares about me." His wife added, "He is a grumpy old man, who is extra grumpy because his leg hurts." I replied, "This is the ER. No one comes when they are having a good day." They both chuckled and he proceeded to tell us about his symptoms. The patient looked at us and said, "You are weird. Why are you listening?" So I told him, "That is the only way we can figure out what is wrong and get you the appropriate help."

Once he realized we were there to listen, he started to talk. And we listened. He opened up about why he was so upset about the care he had received from the medical field up until this point and why he was so upset with life. He had been shuffled around from one doctor to the next and received no answers. He felt the doctors were not listening to his concerns and were just sending him to the next office when they found no answers. They didn't care about him. So why talk here when no one listened elsewhere? The person that took him to all these appointments was his only grandson. He feuded with his son, but his grandson took care of him. He loved his (grand)son like no other. In the weeks just before he came to visit our ER, his only grandson committed suicide.

Just taking a few minutes to listen to his story completely, changed the atmosphere inside the patient's room. He went from being labeled as a violent patient, to a mourning grandfather who was in pain — something we all understood. We were able to get him the care that he needed and he felt that someone finally "listened."

Nurturing and Growing the Future

Suzanna Joy Bell BSN, RN, CCRN

Chantilly, Virginia, USA

It has long been said that nurses eat their young. I have been working in a pediatric ICU for over eleven years now, starting as a new grad. I've seen several generations of brand new nurses come and go; some do well, some don't. To be honest, I was one of the ones that took a while to find my groove, so my empathy naturally lies with the late bloomers.

A few weeks ago, I was on a shift where I was the resource nurse, with a very light assignment, and our admission nurse had less than two years of nursing experience, and was about four months off orientation. A rapid response was called from the pediatric floor on a 20-month-old girl. I went to check on our admission nurse, and make sure the room was ready. As the patient was brought in, I stayed and helped her with admission tasks. Neither she nor I ended up leaving the room. This little girl's care escalated so quickly that we ended up doing over an hour of CPR during a bedside surgical procedure before the night was over. This was the first code that our admission nurse had experienced on our unit.

Our team successfully stabilized this little girl before shift change, and as we reported off to the oncoming nurse, I could read pure exhaustion on my colleague's face. I told her she did a good job passing me meds. I hugged her, and told her to go home and get some rest. I did the same.

When I woke up, I wrote her an email to check on her and to tell her how much I appreciated and admired her willingness to jump feet first, into this difficult and traumatic situation. I let her know that it is still hard for me sometimes, even a decade later, and I reassured her that I was available, anytime she needed to talk or process. She replied that she appreciated my reaching out, and she shared with me that the shift had been one of her hardest. She said she was grateful for my presence and support, and that she'd learned a lot.

It has long been said that nurses eat their young. Let's break that tradition. We should be nurturing our young. The young are the future of nursing. Let's do better for

our sacred profession. Let's do more than survive.
Let's thrive.

Relax and Let Go

Maureen Holt RN, BSN, CHTP
Woodbridge, Virginia, USA

One day on my unit, a coworker's patient was in the process of dying. She was experiencing labored breathing with respiratory stridor. It pained me to hear her in such distress. I volunteered to do Healing Touch and went and introduced myself to her sister. The sister was very upset and sobbing, however, she agreed to let me do Healing Touch. I had the sister sit on the couch as I began to do a technique called Chakra Spread which was developed by a hospice nurse. It involves gently spreading the chakras as you pass over the body three times. As I was beginning the second pass, it suddenly became quiet. The patient had died. I glanced at the sister who was not yet aware. I continued a few more passes, from head to toe, finishing the Healing Touch. When I was finished, I went to the head of the bed and gently told the sister that the patient was gone. She jumped up and said, "Thank goodness she no longer has to suffer." I hugged the sister and stayed with her for a little bit. I feel that the Healing Touch helped the patient to relax and let go.

"Do what you do, Carole. Do it again."

Carole Bergin RN, CHTP
Arlington, Virginia, USA

He was known on the unit as a steely, somber patient. His nurse asked for him to receive Healing Touch. She wasn't certain he would accept, but felt it was worth asking him. His pain was chronic and unrelenting. Pain management was only providing fair relief and still in process. It was just not an optimal effect at this time. Finding the effective combination of medication was yet to be determined. His medications would need more tweaking to reap full benefit. His nurse cautioned me that he was ex-military and that he suffered from PTSD.

Upon entering his room, I observed a small burly man without a smile. I explained my purpose in visiting him was to offer a Healing Touch session. I continued with a brief description of the intervention. To my surprise he accepted the session. His main complaint was that he could not rest because of the pain. My thought was to provide him an intervention that produces relaxation. Relaxation is the key to pain and anxiety management. Because of his PTSD history, I was concerned about actually touching him in any way. I asked him if I could touch him and he gave me consent.

I proceeded with the intervention. As I worked with him I sensed no resistance to light touch used in the intervention. It was difficult to "read him" during his session, since he was so still. Was he dozing off into a sleep state? I could not tell. After the session, his conversation became more animated than initially noted. I did not expect the enthusiasm from such a self-contained persona. He expressed that he felt such peace during the session. He said I ought to provide this Healing Touch to the veterans with PTSD. He was so impressed with the session. The next time I was on duty, he requested another session. He said he had not slept like he did after that previous session in quite some time. He said, "Do whatever you do, Carole. Do it again." As I provided Healing Touch, he dozed off.

It was so fulfilling and an honor to be able to give this patient some moments of peace and rest. He had given so much of himself to each of us through his military service. He was discharged after that day, but I will always remember him.

Changing the Culture with the Caritas Process of the Month

Janet Thomas RN, MSN/MBA-HC, NE-BC
Redwood City, California, USA

Our Chief Nursing Officer adopted Jean Watson as our nursing theorist and based our nursing practice model on Jean Watson's Caritas Processes. Several nurse leaders were sent for the six month Caritas Coach certification (CCEP) course, including the outpatient nurse manager for our hem/onc infusion center.

I heard about the work, and signed up for the four week online course where I was first exposed to caring for oneself, in order to care for others, and the message resonated with me. This felt to be what nursing is all about, in a medical world that has gotten exceedingly complex with technology changing everything about how we care for our patients.

I was so profoundly moved by the work, that I immediately introduced the Caritas Processes as a standing agenda topic on our unit. I started with one multi-disciplinary operations meeting where we had physicians, nurse practitioners, nurses, medical assistants and schedulers. I'd summarize the Process and have one or two people read the few sentences on the Process. Then we would speak to what it meant to us. I then took it to our ambulatory shared governance meeting, and then introduced it into the RN coordinator meeting and it became easy to insert it into a standing agenda topic in even the medical assistant and scheduler's staff meetings.

At our organization we have a 'Readiness Topic of the Month,' that allows our staff to stay focused and on track for regulatory compliance. I thought — Wouldn't it be amazing to have a picture depiction of each Caritas Process, with some brief text speaking to the process as a visual aid?

I joined forces with the outpatient hem/onc infusion center nurse manager, who had just obtained her Caritas Coach certification, and we designed the 'Process of the Month.' We started with Caritas Process 1 in January, and have followed it all the way through the 10th Process for next month. Merian read the "Caritas Process of the

Month," at her daily nursing huddle, and I continued to introduce it as a standing agenda item during meetings. There has been a positive shift that is palpable during our meetings, after the reading of the Caritas Process at hand. Where we might have been mired in past grievances and swirl; we now shift to a proactive mindset with the patient restored to front and center.

Our hospital obtains magnet designation this year. I don't know that we could have achieved this, without the infusion of Caritas Processes into our culture. Thank you Jean Watson for turning on our light of knowing.

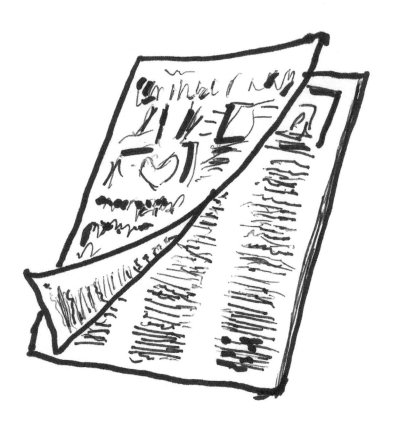

Caritas Process 9

Reverentially assisting with basic

needs as sacred acts, touching

mindbodyspirit of others;

sustaining human dignity.

In the Moment with a Little Angel

Melody Blomquist RN
Highland, Utah, USA

One cannot truly be fully invested in a caring moment without being mindful of the actual moment, and taking in all that is involved in the moment, not only for the self, but for the others that are involved. The Vietnamese Monk Thich Nhat Hanh gave the example of the sheet of paper, and all that is involved with the sheet of paper: its making, its existence, its purpose and fulfillment as what it is. When we translate that to the caring moment that Watson discusses, we see not just the person we are caring for, but all that goes into the making, existence, and purpose of our patient, and ourselves. We all have multiple parts in the ripple/pond. Sometimes we are the stone, and sometimes we are the ripple. So it is with those we care for when we come together for a caring moment.

Describe one instance in a professional setting when you felt mindful caring influence at work. How did it impact the situation?

I had an infant with a very hard beginning and some very special needs who was not at the time, wanted by anyone in particular, and had no home. I allowed myself to be completely involved with this patient, not just 'doing cares kindly,' but speaking with the patient throughout the night, during cares 'eye to eye,' laughing and enjoying every moment that we had together.

A coworker commented, "You are so tender with the patient." What was so impactful was that, though I didn't realize I was being watched, and even though the comment was not particularly important as far as recognition goes, I recognized (because of the comment), that I was totally in the moment with the patient, and that it was important to me personally to be so committed to the welfare of the patient, and the patient's happiness, comfort, and potential. I felt like I really loved and cared for and about my patient.

This is what keeps me in Nursing

Candy Stern Hamacher BSN, RN, CCRN

Waterbury Center, Vermont, USA

I have been a Registered Nurse in Intensive Care Units for over twenty years. When a patient is admitted, it is usually the worse day in the lives of not only the patient but also of his or her family. Out of the seemingly countless cases I have participated in over the years, one in particular crystallized for me the concept of patient centered care in my practice.

Mike was a young man of around twenty-five years who, accompanied by his parents, was directly admitted from his doctor's office to the intensive care unit with worsening respiratory failure. They wore looks of wide-eyed disbelief; in shock that a doctor's visit could land them in an ICU fighting for Mike's life. I quickly learned, during my Nursing Admission Assessment, that Mike was an immensely private person who nevertheless had a wide circle of friends in addition to his three siblings and large extended family. Only his parents knew that he was Gay, and now he requested that they keep this information to themselves alone. He could recall only one unprotected sexual encounter. All previous HIV tests were negative until he arrived in the ICU with full-blown AIDS.

Mike's Infectious Disease physician was the only one I knew, who had worked with AIDS in the 1980s, when virtually everyone died. I had been a young nurse at the time, far removed from this horrible disease and its devastation. Within hours Mike's respiratory status decompensated almost catastrophically. He had several spontaneous pneumothoraxes, requiring four emergent chest tube placements to save his life. Multiple IV sites were established to infuse massive amounts of sedation and powerful anti-retroviral medications from a wall of twelve IV pumps. Tubes were placed in his nose to pump gastric contents out and oxygen in to his lungs, to control his breathing. A tube was placed in his rectum to contain the massive, ever present amount of diarrhea that had eaten away at his skin causing it to bleed spontaneously. Mike's body became covered with the tools to save his life leaving little recognizable of a human body. His parents remained at his bedside constantly.

The next day I attended rounds with the attending Critical Care Physician and the team of residents, interns and medical students. The attending physician was unsure if Mike would survive the day. I interrupted him to say, "We need to include his parents in this discussion." One of the Residents answered with great authority, "No, that mother is not ready to hear this." I incredulously countered, "No parent is ready to hear his or her child is going to die. We are morally obligated to let them know what we are thinking. It is unfair to discuss this without his parents awareness." My words were met with stony silence. But after the meeting, the attending physician arranged with the social worker for Mike's parents to meet with the entire team in the afternoon.

I was present. Mike's parents looked shell-shocked. His mom's face was red and swollen from crying. The attending physician said, "Your son is so sick, I do not know if he will make it through the day." Mom repeated his words, but it was clear to all of us that she did not comprehend what was said to her. The physician again said: " I do not know if he will live through the next 12 hours." Both parents began to cry. Mom was unable to speak. Dad spoke for both of them. "You are saying that we need to notify our family about his impending death?" It was both a statement and a question as he looked to me. I nodded my head and softly stated,"Yes." They asked for some time alone. As we all left the room, I told his parents that I was returning to Mike's room and would answer any questions or help with any follow-up they required. They did not have any questions. Mom and Dad later that afternoon made the decision to call friends and family to inform them of Mike's poor prognosis, even though it would inevitably lead to the disclosure of his sexual preference.

The next day, I went from caring for one incredibly sick young man to directing traffic. There were almost thirty family and friends that stopped what they were doing, and arrived at this young man's bedside. An uncle flew his private plane up from Long Island as soon as he received word. Multiple family members and friends drove overnight and arrived in the middle of the night, with only the clothes on their back and coffee cups in their hands. Overnight, Mike's fraternity brothers' flew from the West coast or drove from multiple points on the East Coast. Most of the brothers were engineers. When they went in the room, they focused on machinery and the monitors and not on the frail, medically sedated, cachexic, dying body that was now covered with tube and wires masking their friend under the technology. They asked endless questions about the waveforms on the monitor which I answered. They proceeded to explain the physics of the waveforms and the internal working of the monitors to me.

Soon Mike's parents took me aside and told me that they were going to get some coffee and allow the "brothers" to spend time with Mike. The small ICU room filled with over twenty tall young men. They phoned Mike's two fraternity brothers that were unable to attend and, using the speakerphone option, placed the phone on Mike's chest. I was startled to hear the room fill with angry male voices, both from the phone and the men present. They were angry because he did not trust them. They demanded to know why he would not want his parents to tell them he was so sick because they all would have been here days ago. At this point, I left the room in order to give them privacy.

Outside the room, one of my colleagues came up to me and asked if I thought it was prudent to leave twenty frat boys in the room with the patient. I tried to sound confident when I responded, "What are they going to do? Kill him? He is already dying." The reality was that I sounded more confident than I felt. Did I do the correct thing to leave a dying man with twenty frat boys and a liter bag of narcotics infusing into his central line? Would the anger erupt into something more? What if he died when I was not in the room? What would his parents say? My supervisor? I trusted the instincts developed over my many years of nursing. I shut the door and let them visit in private. I believed these devoted friends who dropped everything to come to the bedside of a dying friend deserved time alone to say good-bye.

The atmosphere in the room went from angry to party-like. I returned to Mike's bedside and his friend's recounted stories about him. They spoke of his terrible taste in music and his love for expensive booze. They imitated his awful dance moves to everyone's amusement. One of them took me aside and said, "You don't know Mike... he will die trying, but he will always try." The room full of machines, pumps and technology; now had additional coats, laptops and backpacks piled everywhere. The frat boys draped themselves on windowsills, counters, chairs and floor. They turned the sterile, technology ridden ICU room, into a warm familial place where twenty-something year old guys hung out listening to rap music.

Mike remained very ill for over a month. Around week 5, he suddenly turned the corner and made great gains in under a week. His ICU stay was followed by a 1 day Rehab stay. He called his parents after one night at rehab and told them to come get him or he would hitchhike home.

Mike is the only person I have cared for in 20+ years of ICU nursing that was this sick and lived to walk out of the hospital. This experience cemented my belief that acute illness is not just a patient experience, but also a family and friend experience. As professionals, we can use our skills with drugs and technology. Patients have lives and a support system before they become acutely ill. It is our role as nurses to incorporate the support system into our plan of care. I repeatedly told his mom: "If it is good for Mike, then it is good for me. If it is bad for Mike, then it is bad for me."

Unit Grandpa

June Souaya BSN, RN

Alexandria, Virginia, USA

We had a patient for about 3 months who was nonverbal with a sweet countenance. As he had no family we quickly adopted him as our "Unit Grandpa." When a nurse was assigned to this patient, she/he knew it was going to be a good day, despite the effort it would take to care for him. He had such a calming presence on the unit, always greeting people with a smile. He had been found down in his home, covered in feces with a broken arm that had never healed correctly. Clearly traumatized, his eyes would widen, the color would drain from his face, and he would cling to the nearest person when it was time to turn and clean him. Little by little, we got to know him. One clinical technician learned he enjoyed Jimmy Buffett and she got him a Pandora account so he could listen to music. Another nurse discovered he enjoyed dogs, so our therapy dogs came to visit him regularly. When it came time for him to move to a nursing facility as a ward of the state, the unit as a whole pitched in to buy him toiletries, clothes, underwear, slippers, and pajamas. The day he passed, a picture of all the nurses who had taken care of him at Unit Grandpa, was at his bedside. Several staff members went to his funeral and learned he had been a Vietnam Veteran and first responder during 9/11. When I think of Watson's Caritas Processes, I think of my Inova nursing unit, and their devotion to the patient's physical, emotional, and spiritual human needs.

Basic Needs as Sacred Acts

Susan McClanahan BSN, RN, RNC-IPOB

Chantilly, Virginia, USA

On Labor and Delivery we take care of all types of patients with a variety of medical issues. Many days we are assisting in the very happy deliveries of babies. It's a perpetual birthday party! But, other days are quite difficult. Not every family goes home with a happy, healthy baby. Normally, if we have a patient with a fetal demise, we only have the one patient. At times, we have two patients on the floor with fetal demises. One Friday evening, we had an unprecedented four fetal demises. The nurses were searching for any way to comfort the patients and their families. It was night shift and the cafeteria was closed. There was no way to put together a comfort cart of food and drinks. We called the other units, but they also had very little in the way of comfort food. They sent what they had, but we were still short. Panera on our hospital campus is open until midnight. At 2230, we went to Panera and spoke with the manager.

When he learned that there were families on our unit who were in such a sad situation he immediately jumped into action. He began filling up bags with all types of food. In the end, we had more than enough to make four comfort carts complete with coffee. The families were touched by the gesture. And, the nurses felt as though some peace was given to each family. The Panera manager went above and beyond to make sure that the patients and their families were looked after.

The Shower
of Love

A. Lynne Wagner EdD, MSN, RN, FACCE, CHMT,
Caritas Coach
Chelmsford, Massachusetts, USA

The artistry of caring for self and others, when
infused with a conscious loving-kindness, compassion,
authentic presence, and sensitivity to another's frame
of reference, connects two people in a shared heart-
centered, life-altering healing-caring moment (Watson,
2008). This caring moment embodies the ability to
reverently assist a vulnerable person with basic needs as
sacred acts, consciously attending to the person's mind-
body-spirit wholeness (Watson, 2008). This holism,
sustains human dignity and flourishing during health
challenges and beyond. Yet in medicalized objective care
settings, such sacred acts of caring are often missing. I
share two contrasting stories about personal health care
experiences, to dramatically illustrate the differences in
impact and outcomes of non-caring acts that traumatize
and scar, and the caring acts of love that deeply heal

and empower.

I have experienced three episodes of breast cancer in my life. The first was a noninvasive intraductal carcinoma for which I was treated with a surgical wide-excision of the diseased area. The second episode, seven years later, was an extensive reoccurrence in the same breast and required a mastectomy. Emotionally adrift, I worked with my medical team to ensure that my husband could be present with me in the hospital when my primary dressings were removed before discharge. The date and time were arranged and posted in my records. Early on that assigned morning around 5:00 a.m., I was rudely awakened in my dark hospital room by an unknown woman (later identified as an intern) in a white coat, who had already pulled back my blankets and was fiddling with my dressing. Disoriented, I asked, "What are you doing?" She responded, "I need to check your wound and change your dressing." In a flash, before I could protest, the dressing was off. Shocked, I thought, "Okay," and asked for a mirror. She responded, "Why would you want to look at that?" and walked out of the room. Panic and tears were still flowing when my husband and doctor arrived at 10:00 a.m. that day. My doctor was furious and sought the intern. Eventually, with loving support, and an apology from the intern, I was able to look at my chest and begin to heal. But that

damaging trauma of non-caring remains a scar on
my heart.

Again, seven years later, a new invasive cancer was
discovered in the other breast. Another mastectomy was
the best treatment choice, with an additional need to
revise the first mastectomy. A different doctor, a different
hospital. The morning after surgery when I awoke in
pain and anesthesia fog, a young, compassionate nurse
entered my room and sat down next to my bed. She
introduced herself, and asked me how I was feeling,
what I would like to do that day, and what she could
do for me? Out of my fog and despair, I told her I felt
rather disjointed, bruised and beat up. I added as an
afterthought that at home a good hot shower every
morning gets me going. She checked my vital signs, the
occlusive clear dressing that protected my whole chest,
and the four Jackson-Pratt drains, which she emptied.
She added that, "Maybe we can just make a shower
happen today." I laughed at her joke.

An hour later, the nurse returned with an armful
of towels and asked if I was ready to go to the shower
room? "The doctor has approved." I laughed in disbelief.
She said, "Let's get you feeling less bruised." I rode down
the hall in a wheelchair like a queen, towels on my lap.
With help, I undressed and stepped into the shower as
my nurse held the drains. However, I was wobbly and sat

on the shower chair, unable to continue. Instantaneously my nurse had kicked off her shoes and stepped into the shower fully dressed to help me. I tried to protest, but she stood there already wet and asked me to just hold the drains as she tenderly, lovingly washed me. This incredibly healing moment of feeling loved, unjudged, and anointed by the water raining over my body and her sacred act of gentle human touch; soothed my heart and soul with a sense of self worth. In that affirming moment, my mind-body-spirit healing began. She gently dried me and herself, helped me into a clean gown, and comfortably back to bed. I slept deeply, pain-free, for three hours, and my nurse appeared later in fresh dry clothes.

During my three hospital days, my 'Nurse Hero' and I, continued to bond sharing about nursing and caring. She was a new nurse in her first job and so ready to learn and care. We corresponded briefly, but life moved on for the both of us and we lost contact. However, the memory of that healing moment was permanently embedded in my spirit. Amazingly, fifteen years later, I received an unnamed text in response to a nursing conference I was planning, that simply said, "Lynne, is that you?" I knew instantly who it was from, and replied, "Yes. Are you the nurse who cared for me?" Reunited at the conference with tears, she too held the sacredness of our caring moment, forever affirmed in her ways of caring nursing practice. When disillusioned and unfulfilled by hospital nursing a few years into her career, "my nurse hero" had remained true to her beliefs and inner knowing that relational loving-compassionate practice is essential for our profession. I was heartened to learn that instead of leaving nursing, she transitioned to nursing in the community, finding her soul-work again as a healing practitioner.

Reference

Watson, J. (2008). *Nursing: The philosophy and science of caring* (Rev. ed.). Boulder, CO: University Press of Colorado.

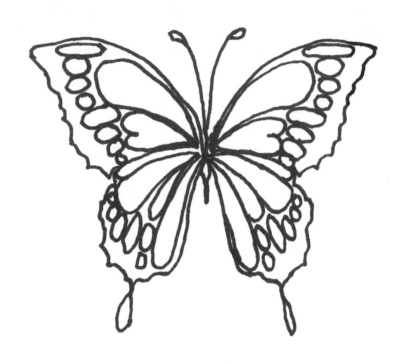

Caritas Process 10

Opening to spiritual, mystery,

unknowns — allowing for miracles.

Being Open to Miracles

Cindy Cannizzaro BSN, RN, HNBC
Toms River, New Jersey, USA

By being open and present to the miracles that
surround me, I have been blessed with many that defy
odds and could only take place with Divine intervention.
I have two areas of practice. Labor and Delivery
and Hospice. I believe that by placing myself at the
beginning and the end of life, brings me to a place that
lends itself to miracles. This miracle happened on the
Hospice unit. This particular night, I wasn't scheduled
to work. I got a call that the unit was becoming busy,
and that they needed a third nurse for the night shift. I
was available, so I agreed to go in. I arrived a little early
to review the patients whom I would be caring for. As
I did this, there was a familiar name. I thought, "It's a
common name, but could it be?" A few years earlier, at a
different hospital, I had worked with an exceptional aide
who became a friend. She had left the position, and we
had lost touch. When I saw her name, I knew the reason

I had been called. She had only arrived in the unit that afternoon. Higher powers were at work, and I was there to care for my friend and comfort her daughter. As I got report, I knew that I would most likely be saying a final goodbye that night. The blessings I was receiving by being allowed to care for her were bittersweet. I went to her room to comfort her family and assess my friend. I asked the family to step out for a moment. I sat by my friend and let her know that I was there. She was unresponsive, but as I talked with her, her breathing changed ever so slightly, letting me know that she knew I was there. I comforted her, assured her that I would be there for her daughter. I then gently bathed her and applied lotion to her dry skin. As I cared for her, I felt honored to have been chosen to be there. When I went to bring her family back in, her daughter had arrived. When she saw me, she fell into my arms and cried. She said she was so glad that I was there, and not a stranger caring for her mother. The family embraced my care knowing that, not only was I her nurse, but her friend as well. The night was peaceful. Friends and some family went home for the night. When everyone who stayed left the room, I sat with my friend and assured her that her family was sad, but okay, and that it was okay for her to rest. Again her breathing changed and she took her last breath with me holding her hand. I stayed with her for a short time, repositioned her and took away all the equipment, and went to comfort her family and bring them to her. There can be no doubt that I was called that day to care for her. Yes I had another patient, but my purpose that night was to comfort my friend and give her permission to go. The blessings that I received that night cannot be described. I was then, and I always will be, open and present for the mystery and the miracles surrounding me in my life.

Race to the Finish Line

Kelli Stangel RN, BSN, CHPN
Spokane, Washington, USA

Because I work with clients at the end of life, so much of what transpires with the client and their Maker after they are unresponsive, is a mystery. I can't ask them what they are thinking, feeling, or hearing. I can provide reassuring touch, whisper in their ears, and watch for nonverbal signs of discomfort, agitation or anxiety; but the mystery of death and what transpires at that moment remains just that... a mystery. I often tell loved ones as well as new grads/hospice nurses, that no one has come back to tell me what that moment is like, the moment of death. I don't know. Which means the person dying does not know either, as they are moving through the process for the first time. I believe it is such a personal and intimate time that others are not to be privy to it. I'm okay with that, as I want that type of privacy when it is my turn. But I have observed some pretty amazing things over the years. One particular occurrence sort of represents all the others in this theme of, "Privacy, please."

I was a floor nurse at the time, caring for a woman who had nine adult children. All nine were at bedside, most with spouses. All the time. Night and day. Around the clock. Never leaving. They used her bathroom for showers, toileting, etc. They stayed in the room during care and repositioning. Did I mention they never left the room? They were wonderful kids, and shared with me how their mom had been widowed early after the ninth child was born, and how she had raised them by herself. They described what a dedicated and involved mom and grandmother she had been. I was blessed by their stories of their childhood and how their mom was the definition of caregiver, other focused and unselfish. This beautiful woman lingered in an imminent state for days on end.

The family began to get vigil weary, as the sprint to get her to the Hospice House turned into a marathon. I spoke often to them about the need to take a break, walk around, smell different smells, hear different sounds; to "normalize" their existence, as the inside of a hospice room doesn't exactly represent normal life. After many days, they started taking turns but still there was a child in the room at all times and as she got closer to her final breath, the room filled again with all nine children. For some reason, on one particular day, I again encouraged them all to step out for the brief minutes it took us to reposition her. To my surprise, they abided. Ladies and gentlemen, I have never seen a woman sprint toward the finish line as fast as this beautiful soul did that day. As soon as the door shut and it was just the client, myself and the HNA, her breathing changed, her skin color changed, and you could almost see her resolve to make her final escape without the watchful eyes of her children. What I gleaned from her is that she wanted privacy. She probably hadn't had any for decades, and that moment was the one moment worthy of not sharing with her children. We were able to get the family back in the room for her final, and I mean final, breath, but I had to smile believing we gave her one moment of privacy and she utilized it to the fullest.

I have seen clients pass when family have stepped out of the room for a cup of coffee, or simply walked into the bathroom in the room to wash hands. I believe it is intentional and, to me, it makes the moment of death all the more mysterious and miraculous.

"Not on my shift"

Joy Shepard PhD, RN-BC, CNE, CDP

Greenville, North Carolina, USA

This is one of my favorite topics. In my personal life and professional nursing practice, I have witnessed many mysterious and miraculous events, illustrating Caritas Process 10. I will take the opportunity here to relate a notable example.

This miracle involved a previously healthy 40-something year old woman who had come down with a deadly fungal pneumonia. She was sedated and on a ventilator with multiple intravenous lines and tubes connected to her deathly ill swollen body. This particular pneumonia was attacking young healthy people, causing critical illness or death within days. These deleterious health events occurred after Hurricane Floyd flooded and overflowed the hog lagoons in some areas of our state, releasing horrible toxins in the land and air. In her case, the prognosis was very poor and she was beyond maxed out on every pressor known to man just to keep her systolic blood pressure barely hanging in the low 80s range.

As I started my night shift, the pulmonologist in

CARING: A PASSAGE TO HEART

charge of my patient breezed right by me with a flock
of residents in tow. Without even acknowledging me,
he stood over my patient's bed (there were no family
present), and made a pronouncement of imminent
death over my patient's near lifeless form. "She will be
dead by midnight," he smugly proclaimed, then exited
just as quickly as he had entered without any further
communication. I thought to myself (as indignation rose
within me), "Not on my shift!" In this case, it was a sense
of indignation (not compassion) that activated the gift of
healing within me.

As a Christian, I believe in the ancient practice of
laying on of hands to impart healing energy or other
beneficial spiritual gifts. The Apostle Paul wrote about
this practice, "Do not neglect the spiritual gift you
received through the prophecy spoken over you when the
elders of the church laid their hands on you" (1 Timothy
4:14). As I felt the gift of healing and a burning sense
of faith rise up within me, I went over to my patient's
bedside and laid hands on her. I rebuked death and
proclaimed in Jesus' name that she would live and not die
and walk out of this hospital! I actually felt healing virtue
flow out of me and into her body. Then, something
truly miraculous occurred. Almost immediately, her
blood pressure began to rise. The moment of prayer
was the turning point; she improved steadily afterwards

throughout the night shift. In the wee AM hours, the flock of residents returned and were truly startled to see this patient still alive and actually improving! Excited, they began to write new orders for her as it looked to them that she may actually live. Indeed, she not only lived but actually walked out of that hospital room many days later.

You Were Right

Emily Barr MSN, CPNP, CNM, Caritas Coach,
PhD Candidate
Denver, Colorado, USA

I was working in infectious diseases and was told about a critically ill little girl who was in the ICU. They believed she had influenza and she was no longer breathing on her own. It turns out the little girl also happened to attend the same church as we did, so I knew her family. This was many years ago, but I will never forget it. The child was so ill, and her heart was failing so they had started her on ECMO. They put her on the heart transplant list and considered moving her to a larger hospital. She was experiencing severe rhabdomyolysis and her kidneys were shutting down. She developed compartment syndrome and needed bilateral fasciotomy on her legs. At this point I asked the attending physician what she thought the prognosis was, and she looked at me and paused, and then told me that she was not going to make it.

My heart felt so heavy. That afternoon I visited the family, but only briefly because I wanted them to know I was available, while at the same time, respecting their space. I told them that I believed she would run again one day. I also remember that I felt a little foolish after I said it, almost as if it wasn't me speaking. Because with her legs split wide open, and waiting for a heart transplant, it was hard to see that future and have that hope.

When you walk into an ICU you can feel the crowds of angels. Even when you are alone with your patient, you never feel alone. There is so much important work happening in the space between life and death. As I left, I prayed for a miracle. I went home and we prayed at dinner and again before bed. And I walked into work the next morning expecting to hear she was either transferred to another hospital or no longer with us, but the pastor from our church was outside her room and told me, "She is alive, and awake. I sat at her bedside praying and around 1 AM one chamber of her heart started working, then a little while later another chamber and by the morning her heart was pumping on its own. Even her kidneys are starting to improve. It's a miracle." The doctors and nurses all agreed that there was no other explanation for her miraculous recovery. She spent months in the hospital learning how to walk again and a year later her mom sent me a card with a photo of her beautiful daughter running during a field day at school with the caption, "You were right."

"I'm in Charge
of Living"

Lorre Laws PhD, RN, Assistant Professor
Tucson, Arizona, USA

Today I will share a story about allowing mysteries to unfold into miracles. In 2010, my then seventy-year-old mother was diagnosed with ovarian cancer, staged at III-b. My parents and I have a very healthy relationship, with all family members communicating transparently, directly, and honestly.

This. Is. Everything.

After navigating the shock of the diagnosis, the debulking surgery, and the first highly invasive round of chemo, we decided to have another "let's get real" conversation. We discussed all-things-end-of-life and quality-of-life. It was decided that we'd make decisions that optimized Mom's quality of life. She declared she'd rather have higher quality with fewer years. My mom's perspective?

"God's in charge of the clock. Dr. ___ is in charge of the cancer. I'm in charge of living."

This one statement became the overarching paradigm of how my mom and our family would live with a cancer diagnosis. There's no fight, no battle with cancer. Rather, there's an earnest surrender to the is-ness of the situation. There's an intention complemented by thoughts and action that position my mom for healing (and, curing, should that become possible), fully living life — in her way, on her terms.

The sequelae of events that followed cannot be explained solely by science (and I'm a scientist!). Mom has an excellent academic-medicine-affiliated oncologist who is also a researcher. Mom has been in two clinical trials, with varying degrees of success. In the first trial, she was the oldest participant and the only one for whom the trial drug was successful; buying her an additional three high quality-of-life years. The second trial resulted in a minor stroke (one of the known side effects of this agent), and so she was un-enrolled from the protocol.

There were many traditional chemotherapy protocols. We've been told three times "This is the last drug available. After this, we'll continue with palliative measures."

Each time the cancer figured out the chemo agent, a new drug was approved... three times.

We're now into immunotherapies, which are generally not very effective for ovarian cancer. We know that cancer will eventually win, or they will keep her alive long enough for something else to be the cause of death (as it is for all of us). We don't concern ourselves with the "what ifs," focusing instead on the richness of the present moment, quality of life, attending to cancer while not making it central in our lives, and being open to miracles and mysteries.

Even without cancer, being open to unknowing, mysteries, and miracles is a beautiful way to live, and is consistent with the teachings of Thich Nhat Hanh, Jean Watson, Eckhart Tolle, among others. Life truly is an adventure. Resist nothing, accept everything, and enjoy the ride...

Meet Me in Paris

Mary Pepin RN
Cranston, Rhode Island, USA

I have worked at Women and Infants Hospital for thirty years. I am a registered nurse with most of my tenure spent in Oncology. Currently, I work in the float pool which means I am trained and skilled in four areas of nursing: Oncology, High-risk Pregnancy, Emergency Room, and Mother-Baby Units. I believe I was called to the float pool so that I would meet Erica and follow her journey through each unit that I am qualified to practice in. As she progressed through each of these units, her care was quite complex.

When I first met Erica, she was 32 years old, 24 weeks pregnant and had received the diagnosis of metastatic stage 4 breast cancer. Immediately upon meeting, she moved me both personally and professionally. Because of my experience taking care of her, my perspective on life changed. She was open and accepting of the many modalities that were incorporated into her care. In addition to the Western medicine that we practice, she expected those who cared for her to adhere to her beliefs. This was difficult for some caretakers. She valued spiritual care and the holistic approach to treatment. We prayed together, we used essential oils, and she was insistent that only natural products be used on her body. Whenever she was preparing to receive any stressful treatment, she would request to have Christian music playing and it had to be close to her ear to help her with the stress and pain that the procedure caused her. I now have a profound fondness for this music — something that I never had in my life.

Erica became my daily assignment which was such a blessing. I was privileged to work with her and her husband, Josh, as well as her entire family. Because I worked 12-hour shifts, I was there for her three meals a day. I would bring my own food, and she would always ask, "What's on the menu today?" I have fond memories of sharing meal time with Erica. I would set up her meal, using sheets for a tablecloth, and I would place a flower in the center of her over-the-bed table. Then we would close our eyes, pretending we were somewhere else. Most of the time, the visualization took us to a small café in Paris, and this soon became our very favorite place. At times, I would bring in food from other cultures so we could experience the world from her room as she was too ill to go home. I now plan to visit Paris in 2020. I will find that cafe we spoke of.

When Erica delivered her daughter, the medical staff

at Women and Infants worked together for the best possible outcome. The tone in the operating room that day was one of total cooperation and determination. Because I had never worked in the operating room, I felt extremely anxious about it. The staff was very supportive and made it possible for me to meet the challenge. My assignment was to be there for Erica while she received anesthesia. I could see that she was getting anxious so I whispered in her ear, "Go to the café in Paris, sit at the table and wait for me. When you're ready I'll come for you." With that said, Erica smiled and closed her eyes peacefully. I knew she was smiling because she knew she would be safe. We were both at peace at that moment as we had been so many times before when we closed our eyes and visualized a beautiful place.

We did not know the outcome of baby Ella, as Erica had had high doses of narcotics, and chemotherapy while pregnant. Baby Ella was delivered via c section, and came out screaming and breathing. She is as courageous as her mother. Erica was intubated and her request was that I place the baby skin to skin and take a photo so that when she woke, she would always have this moment captured. I was able to meet her request.

One of my fondest memories, and I'm sure it was one of Erica's as well, was when she renewed her wedding vows in the Healing Garden at the hospital. She wasn't mobile at the time, but we didn't let that get in the way of her plan. It meant so much to her. I cut her wedding gown up the back and draped it over the front of her beautiful body. Then we wheeled her into the Healing Garden at Women & Infants where she was greeted by fifty people, family and friends. Her presence was angelic, and I had never seen her look happier. This monumental event was a dream come true for her. With her husband, Josh, her children, and her family by her side, she renewed her wedding vows and chatted the day away. Many nurses medicated her throughout the day. I took photos and later presented Erica with an album of the celebration. She made a beautiful bride.

Erica lived for 9 weeks after she delivered, and she made me promise her that I would always stay in contact with her children, her husband and her baby. I have kept my promise attending birthdays each and every year.

Erica touched my life like no other patient has, and when she passed I felt tremendous grief. I felt lost without her in my daily routine. For some time I was unable to visit some of the rooms in the hospital where we had spent time together. Even now, when I go to the room she was in for so many months, I close my eyes and I can sense her presence. I can smell her scent of frankincense oil and I can hear her sweet voice calling to me as she always did at the end of my shift, "I love you, Mary Pepin." And I always responded, "I love you, Erica." We did this daily while she was in the hospital. And I miss it so much.

My grief runs deep, but I find myself turning to the faith that Erica taught me. I have prayed and taken the healing journey of grief. I have had many conversations with my mother who is the closest to me and who recently published her own book about the grieving process. Her advice was to give myself permission to grieve and to use my creativity to memorialize Erica's life in some way. She recommended that I give myself the time it takes to grieve and to connect with people who will listen without judging my feelings. I have formed a great support group of friends and they have guided me through this loss.

It may sound odd when I say that this has been one of the greatest experiences in my life. I lost a patient, with whom I developed a close friendship, and she was very young, but the blessings I received from that relationship are indescribable. And they continue to come to me because Erica's spirit lives on within me. I learned so much from this woman. My spirituality was enhanced by my relationship with her and she taught me to appreciate every moment. I learned to be courageous and kind and to live life with love. I have a better sense of faith now, and I realize how important that is. Sometimes life does not give you who you expect, but accepting what comes your way with courage is possible as a nurse when you have faith. Whatever you believe in, you turn to that for guidance, to get you through. Then you realize that this event was a gift. Erica was a brave woman and my life has changed for the better as the result of meeting her and taking care of her.

I was never comfortable with death because of the implication that the continuity of love ends, and that all we have been no longer exists. With Erica it is absolutely true that her physical body did not survive beyond the experience of death, yet her spirit, her soul, and her essence is what will continue here on earth. She taught me that when my day arrives I now know that I too will live on. I have become a more compassionate vessel of love here on earth because of her.

I love you Erica, and miss you deeply.

Thank you for allowing me to share my journey with Erica and my story.

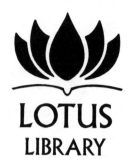

LOTUS
LIBRARY
About Lotus Library

Lotus Library is a publication imprint of Watson Caring Science Institute. Following from the philosophy of Caring Science, Lotus Library aims to encompass and showcase a humanitarian, human science orientation to human caring processes, phenomena and experiences. Our mission is rooted in compassionate care and healing of the mind-body-spirit as one. Our publications exemplify a transdisciplinary approach to sustaining caring/healing as a global covenant with humanity/Mother Earth. Lotus Library provides a forum for nurses and others to give voice to phenomena which otherwise may be ignored or dismissed, celebrating the mysteries of life, death suffering and joy, embracing the miracles of existence.

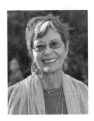

About Jean Watson

Dr. Jean Watson is Distinguished Professor and Dean Emerita, University of Colorado Denver, College of Nursing Anschutz Medical Center campus, where she held the nation's first endowed Chair in Caring Science for 16 years. She is founder of the original Center for Human Caring in Colorado and is a Fellow of the American Academy of Nursing; past President of the National League for Nursing; founding member of International Association in Human Caring and International Caritas Consortium. She is Founder and Director of the non-profit foundation, Watson Caring Science Institute (www.watsoncaringscience.org). In 2013 Dr. Watson was inducted as a Living Legend by the American Academy of Nursing, its highest honor. Her global work has resulted in her being awarded 15 Honorary Doctoral Degrees, 12, international.

As author/co-author of over 30 books on caring, her latest books range from empirical measurements and international research on caring, to new postmodern philosophies of caring and healing, philosophy and science of caring and unitary caring science as sacred science, global advance in caring literacy. Her books have received the American Journal of Nursing's "Book of the Year" award and seek to bridge paradigms as well as point toward transformative models, now, and the future.

For further Lotus Library reading visit our online store: www.watsoncaringscience.org/the-caring-store/

CPSIA information can be obtained
at www.ICGtesting.com
Printed in the USA
FSHW020240280521
81793FS